THEORY AND PRACTICE
IN MEDICAL ETHICS

THEORY AND PRACTICE
IN MEDICAL ETHICS

Glenn C. Graber

and

David C. Thomasma

Continuum · New York

1989

The Continuum Publishing Company
370 Lexington Avenue, New York, N.Y. 10017

Copyright © 1989 by Glenn C. Graber and David C. Thomasma

Printed in the United States of America

Library of Congress Cataloging-in-Publication Data

Graber, Glenn C.
     Theory and practice in medical ethics / Glenn C. Graber and David C. Thomasma
        p.   cm.
     Includes index.
     ISBN 0-8264-0423-5
     1. Medical ethics.   I. Thomasma, David C., 1939- II. Title
     [DNLM: 1. Ethics, Medical.   W 50 G728t]
R724.G75   1988
174'.2--dc19
DNLM/DLC
for Library of Congress   88-39396
                                             CIP

Of one thing we may be sure. If inquiries are to have substantial basis, if they are not to be wholly in the air, the theorist must take his departure from the problems which men actually meet in their own conduct. He may define and refine these; he may divide and systematize; he may abstract the problems from their concrete contexts in individual lives; he may classify them when he has thus detached them; but if he gets away from them, he is talking about something his own brain has invented, not about moral realities.

John Dewey and James Tufts,
Ethics (New York: Henry Holt & Co., 1908)

Contents

This book is dedicated to Edmund D. Pellegrino, M.D.,

educator, clinician, philosopher of medicine, medical ethicist, consultant, and friend,

for his leadership in urging philosophers to work in tandem with physicians in the clinical setting, and physicians and clinical ethicists to consider the philosophical and humanistic basis of this healing enterprise.

And to our wives and families for their constant and loving support for the loss of time together they sustained by both our clinical immersion and joint theoretical reflection.

ACKNOWLEDGEMENTS

We are indebted to our secretaries Kathy Dylan, Kay Cahill Scarano, and JoAnne Immekus for their help in bringing this text to print. Also, the Medical Humanities Program research assistant, J. P. McNulty, deserves our gratitude for his constant help in assembling the background for this text.

INTRODUCTION:

The Problem of Theory and Practice in Medical Ethics

This book is prompted by the authors' reflection and experience in trying to train both medical students and philosophy students in medical ethics. We have found throughout the years that certain questions we had considered about the scope of medical ethics and the role of the medical ethicist were also raised by clinical faculty and by the philosophy students themselves:

- ▶ What should be the role of the medical ethicist on hospital teaching rounds?
- ▶ Should she or he make recommendations about what should be done in a particular case or type of case?
- ▶ If so, how can this approach be defended against the objection that there is no such thing as a moral expert?
- ▶ If making recommendations is *in*appropriate, in what way should we limit the discussion of ethical issues with regard to patient care?
- ▶ In this scenario, what real contribution would ethics or other aspects of philosophy make to clinical decisions about patient management?

Similar questions were raised regarding the objectives of courses.

- ▶ Should courses for medical students merely aim at an intellectual grasp of a variety of positions regarding moral principles, or should they aim at actual training in the *use* of principles by the students?
- ▶ Is clinical experience a necessary ingredient in training philosophy students to teach medical ethics?
- ▶ If so, what should be emphasized by clinicians who supervise this aspect of training?
- ▶ In particular, what criteria should be used to evaluate a philosopher's performance on rounds?

Questions like these forced us gradually since 1973 to develop a philosophy of education regarding medical ethics.[1] Others have also reflected on these issues.[2] However, much philosophical work remains to be done on the questions raised above.

The relation of theory and practice in medical ethics is a difficult theoretical problem, as well as a practical one. It is one that could not have been addressed at all twenty years ago, except perhaps as a footnote to the larger problems of theory and practice in ethics, or more generally still, in all human endeavors.[3]

Before we begin to describe some of the different models of theory and practice, we should explain the terms "theory" and "practice." By "theory," we are *not* referring to the sort of theory *about* ethical language, rules, etc., which dominated philosophical discussion in the third quarter of this century, usually under the label "meta-ethics." The question of the relationship between meta-ethics and normative ethics is an interesting one, which has received attention in the philosophical literature[4] -- but it is not the question with which we are concerned in this book. Instead, we plan to focus on elements of a general, abstract, or theoretical nature *within* ethics (i.e., normative ethics or ethical theory). Beauchamp and Childress have usefully distinguished several levels of generality here.[5] Our emphasis under the heading of theory includes what Beauchamp and Childress refer to as "rules," "principles," and "ethical theories." Thus, we mean by "theory" the embodiment of general and abstract ethical thinking.

The term "practice" includes what Beauchamp and Childress refer to as "judgments and actions," as well as some fairly concrete moral policy statements which they would probably classify as "rules." Hence, by "practice," we mean all forms of conduct by individuals or groups which are capable of analysis in ethical terms, that is, which stem from rational choice about good or evil. These distinctions should become clear in the examples which follow. We will discuss them again in more detail as we go along.

The general question of the relationship between theory and practice, of course, is ancient. It arises for us, as it did for the Greeks and has for every civilization since, because theories influence practice, principles influence conduct, designs influence buildings, concepts influence political realities, ideas influence options. The list of theoretical influences on practical concerns is virtually endless. Similarly the question arises for us because practice influences theory, conduct influences principles, buildings already built and their materials influence future designs, political realities influence social concepts, options persons choose influence their (and others') subsequent ideas. Just as the influence of theory on practice approaches infinity, so too does the influence of practice on theory.

The relation of theory and practice in medical ethics is heightened by one's intellectual prejudice towardsor against deductive ethics, which is often brought into the field of medical ethics from academic training in ethics. We call this an "intellectual prejudice" because it involves assumptions from academic ethics that have not been tested for validity or relevance against the realities of the discipline of medical ethics. In this regard, we detect a growing rift between those who insist on perceiving medical ethics as a branch of applied ethics, those who perceive medical ethics as a reflective branch of medicine itself, and those who hold intermediate positions.[6] Those who teach medical ethics in standard academic settings -- the traditionalists, as it were -- are likely to view those who teach clinically with alarm, because, in their view, one cannot translate ethical reflection into practical advice.[7] The clinical ethicists -- the "New Dealers" -- find themselves more and more impatient with theoretical concerns, especially in the face of so much palpable human suffering. If ethics is about conduct, they might argue, then why should it not be an essentially practical discipline?

Thus, the idea for this book arises from both theoretical and practical concerns. On the theoretical level, it is possible to sketch various positions across a spectrum ranging from the more theoretical or deductive to the more practical or inductive. This task is interesting, and important for critical analysis of the discipline. But also in practice, such a sketch can help to resolve some of the questions raised by medical ethics teaching in the clinical setting. It is pointless to ask which comes first, because theory and practice occur simultaneously. Our own concern, like that of Dewey and Tufts cited in the frontispiece, is that practice be taken as seriously as theory has been by philosophers to date.

The models of theory-practice relation which we shall examine are:

- the application model (chapter 2), which attempts to relate theory to practice in a rigorous deductive fashion;
- the mediation model (chapter 3), which permits minimal independent normative judgment to resolve conflicts of deductively-derived principles;
- the validation model (chapter 4), which begins with a nexus of principles or fundamental values and attempts to develop a policy solution which preserves as many of these elements as possible;
- the determination model (chapter 5), which draws normative force from the categories represented in the practical situation;
- the origination model (chapter 6), which relies entirely on the practice situation for normative elements;
- the virtue model (chapter 7), which puts stress on the kind of person one is to be instead of, or in addition to, the specific actions one is to perform.

We will outline strengths and weaknesses of each of these models, as well as illustrate them in practice through clinical scenarios and specimen arguments. Then, in the final chapter, we will develop an understanding of the relation of theory and practice which avoids the weaknesses of these models and combines their strengths.

To illustrate these models, we will classify particular arguments from authors and policy makers in medical ethics. As with all projects of classification, some distortion may occur. We apologize in advance to our many colleagues should they object to where we have placed them in our schema. Every effort was made to fairly describe positions, but sometimes in terms not of their own choosing. In applying our own labels to their venture, we might have inadvertently misrepresented the scope of their thinking in some fashion. What is most important, we think, is not so much the location of a particular author among these models -- indeed, the reader will find that different arguments by the same author are sometimes placed under different models -- but the structure of the reasoning models themselves and the role these schema can play in clarifying the ways theory and practice are related in medical ethics.

The arguments chosen to illustrate the models deal with a wide variety of issues in medical ethics. Appendix A contains a listing of issues discussed, with chapter citations. This listing readily lends itself to assignments for further research by students. Page references, as well as citations by authors, can be located in the Index.

Glenn C. Graber   *Knoxville, Tennessee*
David C. Thomasma   *Chicago, Illinois*
                               October 1987

Notes

1. Thomasma has published three papers in this regard: David C. Thomasma, "The Possibility of a Normative Medical Ethics," *Journal of Medicine and Philosophy* 5, no. 3 (September 1980), 249-259; "Medical Ethics Training: A Clinical Partnership," *Journal of Medical Education* 54, no. 11 (November 1979), 897-899; and "A Philosophy of a Clinically Based Medical Ethics," *Journal of Medical Ethics* 6, no. 4 (December 1980), 190-196.

Graber has published, with others, a monograph article on the topic: "Extending Humanistic Scholarship Beyond Its Traditional Setting," *Teaching-Learning Issues No. 34* (Learning Research Center, The University of Tennessee, Spring 1977); as well as an essay: "Clinical Medical Ethics Teaching: Objectives, Strategies, Qualifications," in *Clinical Medical Ethics: Exploration and Assessment* (Proceedings of a conference sponsored by the Rockefeller Foundation), ed. Terrence F. Ackerman, Glenn C. Graber, Charles H. Reynolds, and David C. Thomasma (Knoxville: University of Tennessee Inter-Campus Graduate Program in Medical Ethics and University Press of America, 1987).

Graber and two physician-colleagues have published a textbook for medical students which reflects our thinking about this topic: Glenn C. Graber, Ph.D., Alfred D. Beasley, M.D., and John A. Eaddy, M.D., *Ethical Analysis of Clinical Medicine: A Guide to Self-Evaluation* (Baltimore: Urban & Schwarzenberg, 1985).

Thomasma and Edmund D. Pellegrino have addressed some of these issues in their "Philosophy of Medicine as the Source for Medical Ethics," *Metamedicine* 2 (February 1981), 5-11; and "Response to Our Commentators," *Metamedicine* 2 (1981), 43-51, and in their jointly authored book *A Philosophical Basis of Medical Practice* (New York: Oxford University Press, 1981).

2. K. Danner Clouser wrote pioneering articles at the start of philosophers' presence in medical schools on the role of philosophy in medical education: K. Danner Clouser, "Medical Ethics: Some Uses, Abuses and Limitations," *New England Journal of Medicine* 293, no. 8 (21 August 1973), 384-387; K. Danner Clouser, "Medical Ethics: Some Uses, Abuses, and Limitations," *Arizona Medicine* 33 (January 1976), 44-49; K. Danner Clouser, "Biomedical Ethics: Some Reflections and Exhortations," *Monist* 60, no. 1 (January 1977), 47-61; K. Danner Clouser, "Medical Ethics and Related Disciplines," in *The Teaching of Medical Ethics*, ed. Robert M. Veatch, Willard Gaylin, and Councilman Morgan (Hastings-on-Hudson, NY: Institute of Society, Ethics and the Life Sciences, 1973), pp. 38-46, and he has contributed a volume on this topic to the Hastings Center series on ethics teaching and the professions: K. Danner Clouser, *Teaching Bioethics: Strategies, Problems and Resources* (Hastings-on-Hudson, NY: Institute of Society, Ethics and the Life Sciences, 1980), Vol IV in *The Teaching of Ethics*.

Alasdair MacIntyre has argued on at least three occasions that philosophy can make no real contribution to medicine because there are no moral principles upon which a universal consensus about ethical issues could be based: "How Virtues Become Vices: Values, Medicine and Social Context," in *Evaluation and Explanation in the Biomedical Sciences*, ed. H. Tristram Engelhardt, Jr., and Stuart Spicker, (Boston/Dordrecht: D. Reidel, 1975), 97-112; "Patients as Agents," in *Philosophical Medical Ethics: Its Nature and Significance*, ed. H. Tristram Engelhardt, Jr., and Stuart Spicker, (Boston/Dordrecht: D. Reidel, 1977), 197-212; "A Crisis in Moral Philosophy: Why Is the Search for the Foundations of Ethics So Frustrating?" in *Knowing and Valuing: The Search for Common Roots*, ed. H. Tristram Engelhardt, Jr., and Daniel Callahan (Hastings-on-Hudson, NY: The Hastings Center, 1980), 18-35.

William Ruddick edited a monograph containing reflections on the experience of philosophers in the clinical setting at New York University: *Philosophers in Medical Centers* (New York: The Society for Philosophy and Public Affairs, 1980); see also a symposium based on this report, "Can Doctors and Philosophers Work Together?" *Hastings Center Report* 11, no. 2 (April 1981), 12-17.

An examination of clinical ethical methodology questions is contained in *Theoretical Medicine* 7, no. 1 (February 1986), a special issue entitled *Clinical Ethics*, Donnie J. Self (Guest Editor).

Also an important article was published by Ruth Purtilo: "Ethics Consultations in Hospitals," *New England Journal of Medicine* 311 (1984), 983-986.

3. Significant theoretical work on this larger issue is contained in Robert Almeder, *Praxis and Reason: Studies in the Philosophy of Nicholas Rescher* (Lanham, MD: University Press of America, 1982); Mihailo Markovic and Gajo Petrovic (eds.), *Praxis*, Boston Studies in the Philosophy of Science XXXVI (Dordrecht: D. Reidel, 1979); Wolfgang Greive, *Praxis und Theologie* (Munich: Kaiser, 1975); and Hauke Brunkhorst, *Praxisbezug und Theoriebildung: Eine Kritik der Modells entsubjektivierter Wissen* (Frankfurt am Main: Haag und Herchen, 1978).

4. See, for example, William K. Frankena: "On Saying the Ethical Thing," *Proceedings and Addresses of the American Philosophical Association* 39 (1966), 21-42; reprinted in Kenneth E. Goodpaster (ed.), *Perspectives in Morality* (Notre Dame: University of Notre Dame Press, 1976).

5. Tom Beauchamp and James F. Childress: *Principles of Biomedical Ethics*, 2nd ed. (New York: Oxford University Press, 1983), 5ff.

6. Cf. David C. Thomasma, "The Possibility of a Normative Medical Ethics"; Donnie J. Self, "An Analysis of the Structure of Justification of Ethical Decisions in Medical Interventions" *Theoretical Medicine* 6, no. 3 (October 1985), 343-355.

7. Problems with the relation of abstract philosophy to concrete practice were explored in William Ruddick, "Objections to Hospital Philosophers," *Journal of Medical Ethics* 11, no. 1 (March 1985), 42-46; Arthur Caplan, "Ethical Engineers Need Not Apply: The State of Applied Ethics Today," *Science, Technology, and Human Values* 6, no. 33 (Fall 1980), 24-32.

CHAPTER ONE
Definition of Terms

Both novices and cognoscenti encounter a great deal of frustration when dealing with medical ethics; in part, because the usage of various terms has not been made sufficiently clear. Confusion about these terms can easily muddy a consideration of questions regarding the relation of theory and practice. In order to avoid these difficulties, therefore, it is important to spell out at the start the meaning of various key terms we will employ throughout the study. The vocabulary proposed is as follows: "principles," "rules," "axioms," "policies," and "indicated courses of action."

We shall proceed in this chapter term by term. But first consider some initial distinctions which arise from levels of moral reasoning in schema 1a.

We will discuss the research-on-children arguments further as examples of deductive reasoning in chapter 2. At this point the argument is broken out into component parts the more easily to detect levels of argumentation and the relationship between them. In a sense, each of these levels of argument *leads to* the next. Given McCormick's theological emphasis on the doctrine of creation, for example, it is unsurprising to find him focus on a natural-law ethical theory, since this draws upon norms "built into" nature in the process of creation. However, this move is not a strict deductive necessity. One might, for example, move from a theology of creation to a divine-command ethical theory -- using either an argument that employs a creaturely duty of *gratitude* or one that incorporates a notion of divine *ownership*. Similarly, the Stoic proponents of a form of natural law theory unpacked it in terms of different principles than the focus on the common good that McCormick develops.

This schema is based on a logical ordering. Thus it does not capture one key question with which we shall be grappling in these pages -- the issue of *epistemic* ordering. Do we first come to know abstract theories, then principles, and only then derive concrete guidelines from these, or is it epistemically possible to come to know first what is the right thing to do in a specific situation and to justify principles and theories on the basis of these indicated courses of action?

In a sense, then, as an argument unfolds one's theory is entailed in one's meta-ethical belief, one's fidelity to the center of value in one's life and thought, one's principles in one's theory, and so on, down the line. Note also that rules are a step outside an argument,

1a

McCormick-Ramsey Debate About
Non-Therapeutic Research on Children

	McCormick	**Ramsey**
Meta-ethics	Theological Basis: Doctrine of Creation	Theological Basis: Doctrine of Covenant
Ethical Theory	Natural Law - inclination towards community, concept of the "common good"	Covenant-ethics (between persons, under God); *Agape*
Principles	We all ought to bear certain burdens for the common good. (Justice)	a) Respect for Persons - It is absolutely wrong to treat persons as means. b) Benevolence is an expression of *charity*, not an obligation.
Rules	Rule of proportionality: An act must be in proportion to both benefits and principles.	Rule of applicability: Children are persons.
Axioms	Non-therapeutic research on children is justified if a) risk is minimal, b) proxy consent is obtained, c) design, etc. promises benefit.	If consent is impossible, non-therapeutic research is absolutely wrong.
Indicated Course of Action	Project *x* is acceptable.	Project *x* is unacceptable.

a method of interpreting, not only facts with which a case is concerned, but also the progress of the argument itself. Thus axioms may depend as much on one's interpretation rules as on one's principles.

Unless otherwise noted, we shall use the terms to be defined according to this schema and the definitions to follow.

A. Principles

Moral principles express fundamental theoretical norms -- as, for example, Mill's "We ought to maximize the general happiness," or Kant's categorical imperative. The term "principle" comes from the Latin *principium*, a translation from the Greek *arché*, and means a start or beginning. Thus the term also connotes a *source* from which there can be derivations. In effect, then, by calling something a principle, one claims (a) that no more fundamental norm is forthcoming and (b) that from this source (whatever it may be) can be derived certain conclusions. Thus, usage of the term already incorporates a view that principles may entail judgments, or that one may derive certain action-guides which are implied in principles. In short, theory has implications for practice. A fundamental moral principle, like "All persons ought to be respected" is prescriptive.[1] It commands certain actions. As we shall show in chapter 2, there are any number of appropriate "indicated courses of action" which could preserve the moral force of the principle. In this sense, these can be said to be derived from it. But there are also certain actions which would violate the principle, actions such as subjugating a person to another's will. These actions are then proscribed by a prescriptive principle.[2]

However, such implications may not be as direct nor as linear as some moral theorists have suggested. An immediacy of concrete obligations or imperatives entailed in moral principles is assumed by W. I. Matson in his attempt to analyze Kant as a casuist. He says:

> I shall mean by casuistry that species of deductive argument having as conclusion the assertion that a particular person is morally obliged to perform a certain act and having as premises (a) statements of fact about the person and the act and; (b) a philosophical theory of moral obligation, or at least one or more general statements deduced from such a theory.[3]

As Matson supposes, the demand to perform a certain action is, by deductive logic, entailed by the premises, at least one of which is a normative principle. This is the pattern of reasoning we shall call "the application model," and shall examine at length in chapter 2. Matson also notes, parenthetically, although casuistry has received a second, more odious meaning, its analogues such as medicine, art criticism, engineering, and the like, are all honorific professions.[*]

Less specifically centered on personal obligations to perform certain actions is the theory of ethics proposed by Saint Thomas Aquinas, based on Aristotle's *Nichomachean Ethics*. Aquinas proposed that ethical judgment is a quasi-conclusion of a practical syllogism, if one takes ethical judgment to mean the virtue of prudence or practical judgment.[4] Aquinas's argumentation about the relation of moral theory to practice is quite sophisticated. First he tries to establish that the natural law embodies precepts of reason: "The precepts of natural law are related to practical reason in the same way the basic principles of demonstrations are related to theoretical reason, since both are sets of self-evident principles" *(art. 2)*. He then argues, after a discussion of ways in which we may understand the meaning of the term "self-evident," that the first thing that is self-evident or within the unrestricted grasp of the practical reason is the good: "Good is the first thing to fall within the grasp of practical reason -- that is, reason directed to a work -- for every active principle acts on account of an end, and end includes the intelligibility of good" *(art. 2)*.

From these considerations Aquinas is then led to the first principle of practical reason, or in modern terminology, the foundation principle of ethics: "It follows that the first principle of practical reason is one founded on the intelligibility of the good -- that is: Good is what each thing tends toward. Therefore, this is the primary precept of law [natural law]: Good is to be done and pursued, and evil is to be avoided. All other precepts of the law of nature are based on this one, in this way that under precepts of the law of nature come all those things-to-be-done or things-to-be-avoided which practical reason naturally grasps as human goods or their opposites" *(art. 2)*.

The point to be pressed is that the first principle is not necessarily imperative in the casuistic sense claimed by Matson (much less in Hare's sense, to be examined just below); rather the conclusion of the practical syllogism is an action to be done or avoided, not a command to a particular person. In other words, additional steps, such as examining one's values, seeking counsel with others, considering other germane duties, and grappling with other existential considerations, are necessary before a person decides to take such an indicated course of action.

---

[*] Jonsen, among others, has suggested that medical ethics could more properly be considered a form of casuistry because of its close parallel to medical reasoning. Of course, he defines casuistry in a more traditional way than does Matson. These views are left for later consideration in chapter 8.

R. M. Hare insists on the nature of moral judgment as "prescriptive." By this he means, first, that statements in ethics dealing with value and the good must be justified by terms other than an appeal to facts. "It is better to take the train than the plane to Chicago," cannot be justified solely by an appeal to factual matters, such as "You know that you get sick on the plane." The latter justification becomes relevant to the prescriptive only if and when it is conjoined with a norm that one ought (in Hare's view, a "decision of principle") to avoid becoming sick. Justification of prescriptives embodies the "supervenient" character of moral values -- non-ordinary justification.[5] All normative and prescriptive judgments have the same logic in this respect.

Furthermore, for Hare, to make a decision of principle is to accept the prescriptive nature of a principle -- that is, to accept the command that flows from it: "Does he or does he not recognize that if he assents to the judgment he must also assent to the command: Let me do x"? This is the way Hare suggests we check on whether a person is using moral language correctly.[6]

However, Germain Grisez and other critics of Hare have argued for distinguishing imperative force from prescriptive. Imperative force is Hare's notion that within moral principles are commands to carry out certain actions, or at least, that from such principles can be derived such commands. Grisez argues that Aquinas did not mean this by his own first principle. Rather, the meaning of precepts in Aquinas's system of thought was that they do not:

> inform us as of requirements; they express requirements as directions for action. The point of saying that good is to be pursued is not that good is the sort of thing that has or is this peculiar property, obligatoriness -- a subtle mistake with which G. E. Moore launched contemporary Anglo-American ethical theory. The point rather is to issue the fundamental directive of practical reason.[7]

Armed with these distinctions, we may further refine the definition of "principle." A moral principle is an ought-statement which may express (or yield) a command about (imperative), a precept towards(prescriptive), or a description of (descriptive) conduct to be done or avoided. A command and a precept are simply different types of prescriptive principles, both distinct from descriptive ones.

The use of principles to describe a body of statements about proper practice, such as the principles of ethical conduct for surgeons formulated by the American College of Surgeons,[8] would then be an improper term. The proper term here might be "standards," rather than "principles." The AMA makes such a distinction in its Judicial Council Proceedings.[9]

Other ethical theorists agree that ought-statements need not always be prescriptive in Hare's narrow sense. Kerner, for example, excoriated Hare for "failing to recognize the total difference" in meaning between imperatives and ought-judgments.[10] Although this charge is perhaps overstated (Hare may *recognize* the difference), the point is well-taken. It is not the case that every ought-statement need reflect specific commands, as we have already shown in Aquinas's analysis.

Although for Hare the difference between ought-statements and imperatives lies largely in the fact that imperatives may not always be universalizable as ought-statements must be, there is a deeper difference as well. Warnock and Foot have both developed the naturalist or descriptive aspect of ethics in direct opposition to Hare. The debate between these camps originates in Hume's claim that ought-statements cannot be derived from is-statements -- the now-famous warning[11] which went largely unnoticed until Moore issued his criticism of what he called the naturalistic fallacy.[12] Ethical intuitionists like Prichard and even emotivists like Ayer, discuss this logical rule (as well as Moore's linguistic rule which he does not distinguish from it) and profess to follow them.[13] Hare is the most explicit in claiming to honor "Hume's rule."[14] Of course what these thinkers interpret the naturalistic fallacy to mean is: (a) that the "ought" cannot be entailed by the "is"; and (b) that there is thus an insurmountable gulf for normative statements, because all ethics is either deductive (in the sense that commands are entailed by moral principles) or defective. As we shall see in the chapters to follow, both these claims can be challenged.

If no description can be used to prescribe, then the purely deductive view of ethics must prevail. All moral principles are thereby rendered either imperative or prescriptive. If descriptive principles *can* be used to prescribe, then some descriptive principles could be employed to prescribe in the sense Aquinas uses when discussing the first principle of practical reason, namely, as a guide or map of appropriate action or actions, without a specific command to any particular individual.

One interpretation of Hume's is-ought passage, which may in fact mean something quite the opposite of Hare's interpretation, is that Hume held, as did many other major moral thinkers, that the "ought" entails a consensus of judgment or the good of the community. As Alasdair MacIntyre argues:

> the notion of "ought" is for Hume only explicable in terms of the notion of a consensus of interest. To say that we ought to do

something is to affirm that there is a commonly accepted rule; and
the existence of such a rule presupposes a consensus of opinion as
to where our common interests lie. An obligation is constituted in
part by such a consensus . . . .[15]

We will rely on this point when developing a biomedical hermeneutics
in a unified clinical ethics theory in the final chapter.

To this view (that principles may include precepts or norms that
sketch the territory for action rather than command it) is added the
observation that Aristotle's practical syllogisms frequently included
wishes, wants or desires in at least one premise, just as Aquinas
argued that the first principle of ethics is not a command to do good
and avoid evil, but a statement of the good found in nature
towardswhich all creatures tend. Hence, MacIntyre continues:

We could give a long list of the concepts which can form such
bridge notions between "is" and "ought": wanting, needing, desiring,
pleasure, happiness, health -- and these are only a few. I think
there is a strong case for saying that moral notions are
unintelligible apart from concepts such as these.[16]

For this and other reasons we hold that principles do not
necessarily directly command action, but that action-guiding commands
could be derived from principles. To speak of imperative principles,
is therefore, to speak of those principles from which such commands
could emanate. The level of principles is generally too abstract for
commands of specific actions. Middle-level principles, axioms, or rules
or some other bridging premises are necessary to develop conclusions
such as "Do this action!" The form such derivations take, as well as
the source of principles themselves, will be the subject of detailed
inquiry in future chapters.

B. Rules

All moral theory rests on a set of beliefs about the way society
and human affairs ought to be run. These beliefs may be religious,
philosophical, political, pragmatic, and/or self-serving. An organized
body of such beliefs is a theory, with second order ideas for its use
and for its testing in human experience. We call these beliefs "rules,"
to distinguish them from either fundamental norms for action, on the
one hand and moral axioms or middle-level principles, on the other
hand. *A rule*, say the "double-effect," *is a guide which stands extrinsic
to the norm and which is employed for interpreting and applying the
normative principle in practice.* A rule is a methodological or
procedural interpretant; whereas an axiom is a substantive, moral
interpretant.

We suggested that by principles we should mean ought-statements expressing a theoretical norm. Examples would be: "Persons ought to be respected" (deontological); "The benefit of all ought to be a greater good than the benefit of a few" (utilitarianism); "One ought to do good and avoid evil" (natural law theory). (It should be noted that there is another non-deductive, virtue-centered natural law theory in which this principle would not have prescriptive force.) Because these theoretical judgments are so general, they require not one type of interpretation but two, axiomatic and nomian, the former corresponding to intrinsic valuation (axioms) and the latter to extrinsic (rules).

The extrinsic interpretant of a principle is a moral rule, what we have termed a "nomian" interpretant, after the Greek word for law. A moral rule assists its users in adjusting the weight of the values represented in principles by interpreting, not their meaning in a particular context, but their applicability relative to other values.[17] The context (which we shall subsequently argue is a moral rule) does not determine the moral significance of an event as much as help prioritize values within that event. In a case contrasting a doctor's responsibility to help patients with their refusal to concur with the doctor's recommendation, a deontological rule might be the categorical imperative. Deciding among competing values, in order to "weigh" respect for persons and the autonomy axiom properly, doctors must act in such a manner that what is done would become a universal law. If they could not will it done to themselves, or others they could imagine, then their plan of action would not be a valid interpretation of the deontological principle.

In the same case, a utilitarian moral rule might be a calculus of benefits to the doctor, patient, and society, under which one could choose that course of action most able to respect as many benefits as possible. Although it has pragmatic overtones as well, this seems to be the position on the nature of bioethics held by Ackerman.[18] If so, then the extrinsic moral interpretant in a utilitarian medical ethics passes no judgment on the strengths of each value as such. Rather, this rule requires a quantitative respect for as many standard values as possible.

A final example would be the "principle" of double effect as an extrinsic interpretant of natural law theory. It is not really a principle as now defined, but rather a moral rule guiding the application of doing good and avoiding evil when good actions may lead to evil results. Among other things, the rule states that the evil result cannot be intended, nor can it directly issue from the action taken.

We hope it is now clear that values, as expressed in judgment-form in principles, are capable of intrinsic and extrinsic interpretation (reassessment, prioritization, weighting, and evaluation).

Intrinsic interpretation is carried out by axioms which make the principle more concrete. Extrinsic interpretation can require making an application of a principle into a universal law, making an application of a principle into a respect for many values, and ruling out an application if it may be misapplied. There are certainly other moral rules as well, but these suffice to clarify their role as application-interpretants in contrast to substance-interpretants (axioms). We shall focus on moral rules at length in chapter 5. This usage of "moral rules" to apply to application-interpretants, of course, differs from Bernard Gert's usage as applicable to precepts.[19]

C. Axioms

Intrinsic middle level principles are required to interpret or give more specific content to moral principles. We call these middle-level principles "axioms." *Axioms state intrinsic moral interpretants of a principle, through which it can be employed and specified in a context.* Following the same order as that used for principles, examples of axioms would be: "Enhancing patient autonomy is a necessary way of respecting persons" (deontological); "Calculating the greatest good for the greatest number of people is a necessary way to enhance the benefit of all" (utilitarianism); "The good in this case is to restore this patient's sense of self-worth" (natural law). There are innumerable axioms which can help refine and specify the principle. Further, axioms from different theories of ethics and medical ethics often can be used to specify principles of other theories. Axioms, then, acquire their meaning less from a meta-ethical theory (as do principles) and more from everyday life. Unlike rules, axioms are not methodological interpretants, but substantive ones. They help focus the point of the moral principle on the matter at hand.

Purely deductive ethical systems, such as those we shall discuss in chapter 2, rely totally on these minor premises to reach commands. Modified deductive systems rely on a number of factors, including these axioms, to reach a guideline for action.

Whatever the considerable merits of approaching medical ethics in a case-analytic fashion, the notion of intermediate principles, or axioms, is clearly demanded as one bridge between the abstract and the usual. John Stuart Mill himself noted:

> Without such middle principles an universal principle, either in science or in morals, serves for little but a thesaurus of commonplaces for the discussion of questions, instead of a means of deciding them.[20]

One of the causes of confusion about ethical terms is the fact that an axiom in one system of ethics might be a principle in another.

Or, a descriptive principle in another system might be regarded as a norm in yet another, and an axiom in a third. For example, if autonomy is regarded as the most fundamental principle in Kant's theory, then beneficence would be at most a normative axiom, a means to carry out respect for autonomous entities. In a utilitarian ethical system, however, beneficence has to be regarded as the most fundamental principle. In another, Aquinas's ethics for instance, the fundamental principle is "Do good and avoid evil," so that respect for persons is a lesser axiom representing an action towardsthe good, and beneficence, ranking higher, is at the center of all human acts.

D. Policies

In addition to principles, rules, and axioms, we will also speak of policies and indicated courses of action. *Policies provide ought-statements which indicate how to resolve conflicts among principles and axioms in certain situations.* The reason that policies are important is that they express more action-oriented resolutions of human dilemmas than do principles. Thus, they are less universal than either moral principles or axioms. A moral policy approach to the resolution of difficulties in medicine admits of a plurality of general but not absolute principles and axioms. It requires a consensus of the community about which values in conflict to protect in a given course of action, in a way parallel to MacIntyre's reading of Hume's ought-statements.

Thus, to use an example cited earlier, a policy requiring that minors consent or assent to medical research performed on them protects their developmental rights, their own welfare, and their growth as autonomous persons, while judging less important in this instance values of family autonomy from state interference, the rights of parents to decide what is best for their children, and so on. The danger of policies is that a "decision" about difficult moral dilemmas in one sphere sets a precedent which may cause problems in another. For example, does giving minors the right to dissent from nontherapeutic research also give them the right to withdraw from experimental therapy which is potentially lifesaving, even though we might question the soundness of their judgment?[21]

Arthur Dyck was one of the first to pay particular attention to the ramifications of moral policy:

> Moral policy refers to that portion of the total ethical enterprise in which whatever is known or believed to be true in normative theory as well as meta-ethical theory is applied to specific moral issues and the methods used to cope with them. Decisions about what is right or wrong . . . are not solely decided, nor ought they be, on the basis of ethical theory per se.[22]

Dyck's suggestion, then, can be a foil to the merely case-by-case resolution of issues, which cannot provide a framework for understanding the relation of moral theory, principles, and axioms to the matter at hand. We shall discuss the role of policies at length, as well as the sort of reasoning which leads to them, in chapter 4.

E. Indicated Courses of Action

An indicated course of action is the conclusion of a practical syllogism. As such it describes what ought to be done in a particular circumstance; even though it does not command this action, considerable effort would have to be made to justify not doing it. The distinction between policies and indicated courses of action lies in the fact that it is not assuredly possible to move from a judgment that x is a morally right or wrong course of action in this specific circumstance, to one that x is a morally right or wrong policy. Beauchamp and Childress cite other factors intervening in the latter judgment, such as the cost and burdens to society or the symbolic value of the law.[23] One can judge that in a particular circumstance abortion is a morally wrong course of action while still holding that legal permission for abortion is good as a social policy because it meets the needs of others not disposed to make the same judgment. An indicated course of action is different from a moral action-guide in that the former is a concrete action to be performed - for example, asking *this* patient for her consent to surgery -- rather than an overriding and general guideline for action (such as, "Informed consent ought to be obtained in all surgical cases").

F. Conclusion

It is helpful to insist on distinctions among stages and between content and methodological axioms while admitting that terms for the stages may be employed differently by other thinkers. For example, a catalogue of component stages in moral reasoning was offered in 1968 by Paul Ramsey:

> Our model of the component stages in moral reasoning can, therefore, be stated as follows: ultimate norm; general principles; defined action principles or generic terms of approval and generic offense terms; definite-action rules or moral species terms; then the subsumption of cases.[24]

Ramsey's listing is useful to underline the confusion caused in ethics and medical ethics by lack of agreement regarding terminology at different levels of moral reasoning, while simultaneously exemplifying the general agreement that stages proceed from more general to more specific. There are identifiable levels, each with different functions. Ramsey's ultimate norm is our moral principle. As we understand Ramsey, his general principles are our rules; his defined action principles, containing words of approval and opprobrium, are our policies. His definite-action rules seem to parallel our axioms. His case analysis includes our indicated courses of treatment.

A summary of terms and relationship discussed is provided by the schema in figure 1.

In this schema, note that we have limited the use of the term "practical reason" to the function of relating principles, axioms, rules, and standards. "Practical judgment" relates axioms and circumstances, both those that are unique and those that are similar to other cases. "Prudential judgment" takes these unique and analogous cases into account in issuing actions to be done. We reserve "conscience" for the judgment that issues a command to a person to perform a specific action. In no way should such a command be misconstrued as present in a general principle, axiom, or even circumstance. Virtue and training do have a lot to do with such commands, however. Nonetheless, from principles can be derived more and more specific axioms, although even these will be influenced by the community's experience, if not in suggesting the principles and regarding them as valid, then at the very least in the formulation of rules for their application. We regard the categorical imperative, the calculus of pleasures, and the "principle" of double-effect in the deontological, utilitarian, and natural law traditions respectively to be just such methodological rules for interpreting the relation of principles (autonomy, utility, and "Do good and avoid evil," respectively) to axioms and circumstances. Finally, note that in our schema, practices have a major impact on axioms. Of course, they would also influence community standards and rules, as shown, as well as create the circumstances and indicated courses of action (not shown).

Figure 1

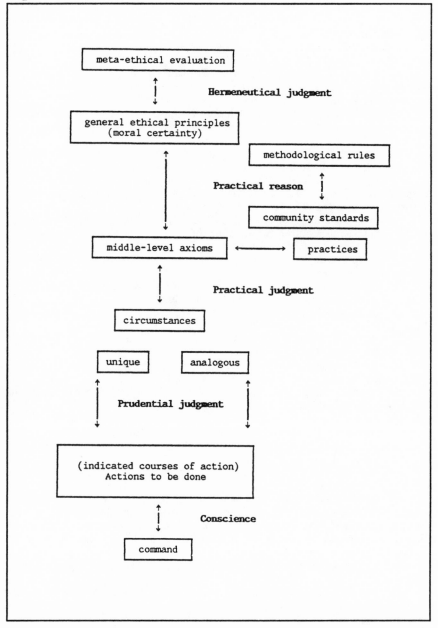

NOTES

1. R. S. Downie, Elizabeth Tefler, *Respect for Persons* (New York: Schocken Books, 1970).

2. David C. Thomasma, "The Basis of Medicine and Religion: Respect for Persons," *Linacre Quarterly* 47 (May, 1980), 142-150.

3. Wallace I. Matson, "Kant as Casuist," in Kant: *A Collection of Critical Essays*, ed. Robert P. Wolff (Notre Dame: Notre Dame University Press, 1968), p. 331.

4. Saint Thomas Aquinas: *Summa Theologiae*, 102, Q. 94, art. 2.

5. W. D. Hudson, *Modern Moral Philosophy* (New York: Doubleday Anchor Books, 1970), pp. 164-167.

6. R. M. Hare, *The Language of Morals.* (Oxford: Oxford University Press, 1952), pp. 168-169.

7. Germain Grisez, "The First Principle of Practical Reason," in *Aquinas: A Collection of Critical Essays*, ed. Anthony Kenny (Notre Dame: Notre Dame University Press, 1976), p. 374.

8. American College of Surgeons: *Statement of Principles*, April 1, 1977.

9. American Medical Association Judicial Council, *Current Opinions* (Chicago: American Medical Association, 1984), §1.01 and §1.02.

10. George C. Kerner, *The Revolution in Ethical Theory* (Oxford: Oxford University Press, 1966), pp. 148-167.

11. David Hume, *Treatise on Human Nature*, §III.i.1, ed. L. A. Selby-Bigge (Oxford: Clarendon Press, 1964), pp. 469-470.

12. G. E. Moore, *Principia Ethica* (Cambridge: Cambridge University Press, 1903).

13. H. A. Prichard, *Moral Obligation* (Oxford: Oxford University Press, 1949), p. 89, 134.

14. R. M. Hare, *Freedom and Reason* (Oxford: Oxford University Press, 1963), p. 108.

15. Alasdair MacIntyre, "Hume on 'Is' and 'Ought,'" *The Philosophical Review* 68 (1959), 457-458.

16. Ibid.

17. Terrence F. Ackerman, "What Bioethics Should Be," *Journal of Medicine and Philosophy* 5, no. 3 (1980), 260-275.

18. Ibid.

19. Bernard Gert, *The Moral Rules: A New Rational Foundation for Morality* (New York: Harper and Row Torchbook, 1973).

20. John Stuart Mill, "Dr. Whewell on Moral Philosophy," in *Mill's Ethical Writings*, ed. J.B. Schneewind (New York: Macmillan, 1965), p. 178.

21. David C. Thomasma, Alvin M. Mauer, "Ethical Complications of Clinical Therapeutic Research on Children," *Social Science and Medicine* 16 (1982), 913-919.

22. Arthur Dyck, *On Human Care* (Nashville: Abingdon Press, 1978), p. 115.

23. Beauchamp and Childress, *Principles of Biomedical Ethics*, p. 12.

24. Paul Ramsey, "The Case of the Curious Exception," Gene Outka and Paul Ramsey (eds.), *Norm and Context in Christian Ethics* (New York: Charles Scribner and Sons, 1968), p. 78.

CHAPTER TWO
The Application Model

The first model of the relation of theory and practice in medical ethics which we shall discuss is probably the most popular and, in a way, the most direct. In this approach, theoretical normative principles are taken as givens. The transition to practice is made through some formal, linear inference or similar method.

A. Examples of the Application Model

(1) The most straightforward form of this approach would be a deductive practical syllogism in which the major premise is a normative judgment and the minor premise is a description of the relevant features of the context of action. For example, Paul Ramsey's position on nontherapeutic research on children[1] can be presented in terms of syllogism 2a.

2a

Normative premise: One ought never to use a person as a subject in nontherapeutic research unless he or she has given free and informed consent to participate.

Description of situation: No young child has given free and informed consent to participate in any nontherapeutic research (because children are *incapable* of this sort of rational decision on their own).

Conclusion: One ought never to use a young child as a subject in nontherapeutic research.

In the terms introduced in the previous chapter, the normative premise is a "middle-level axiom" rather than a foundational principle; the descriptive premise is an axiom of application; and the conclusion is a statement of policy. This reasoning can be extended in both directions through additional syllogisms of the same type. The resultant policy conclusion can be brought down to the level of a specific indicated course of action through a syllogism like 2b.

2b

Normative premise: One ought never to use a young child as a subject in nontherapeutic research.

Description
of situation: The research protocol which Professor Jones proposes to undertake comprises nontherapeutic research on young children.

Conclusion: Professor Jones's protocol ought not to be implemented.

This conclusion offers specific advice for action -- for example, to members of an Institutional Review Board who are reviewing Professor Jones's protocol. The guidance is clear. They ought to refuse to authorize this project.

The moral norm that functions as the major premise of the argument cited initially can itself be derived from an even more abstract moral *principle* in a syllogism like 2c.

2c

Normative premise: One ought to treat each person as an end-in-himself or herself and never merely as a means.

Description
of situation: To use a person as a subject in nontherapeutic research when he or she has not given free and informed consent to participate is to treat him or her merely as a means.

Conclusion: One ought never to use a person as a subject in nontherapeutic research unless he or she has given free and informed consent to participate.

The distinctive characteristic of this model of reasoning is that the normative thrust comes entirely from the major premise. The process of applying the moral principle to the situation at hand involves, not independent normative thinking, but rather reasoning processes of conceptual analysis, classification, and other nonnormative modes of thought. For example, in syllogism 2a cited above, the issue in the minor premise is primarily a matter of conceptual clarification and classification. The question is what counts as "free and informed consent" and whether the reasoning ability of a young child is sufficiently developed that we would say that she or he is capable of giving free and informed consent. Once this conceptual issue is settled, no further normative reasoning is needed to make the transition from the theoretical major premise to the practice-level conclusion of the argument.

This feature is even more obvious in the second of the three arguments cited, Syllogism 2b. The issue here is to determine whether Professor Jones's protocol (a) involves research, (b) involves children as subjects, and (c) is nontherapeutic in nature. Once these issues are settled, the normative conclusion follows automatically and rigorously.

Syllogism 2c is more problematic on this score. To determine whether a certain form of activity involves "treating persons merely as means" may seem to go beyond conceptual clarification and classification and to involve normative reasoning. One will be inclined to judge that the activity at issue *does* involve treating persons merely as means when, and because, they have a "gut feeling" that the activity is *morally wrong*. But this appears to be independent normative thinking which intrudes into the reasoning process at this point. Something similar is involved, to a lesser extent, in the other two arguments. One who has a "gut feeling" that the activity is morally unacceptable will be more inclined to rule that it involves *un*free consent or *un*informed consent or that it does not involve genuine consent at all. In syllogism 2b, one who approves of the research protocol at a "gut" level is likely to urge that it does not involve research as such, or else that the research is therapeutic (at least in part), and thus that it does not fall under the moral rule that forms the major premise of the argument.

The possibility of these normative intrusions into the deductive application of the moral principle to the situation at hand has several implications. First, it shows that the line between this model and the mediation model (to be discussed in the next chapter) is not sharp. Indeed, this is one criticism we make of the application model later in this chapter. It is unlikely that pure deductive application without any admixture of normative mediation is possible. But, second, it is important to notice that in this model of reasoning the normative concepts in the major premise at least function to limit the sorts of normative reasoning which can be interjected.   The focus of the dispute is determined by the normative principle which functions as the major premise.

It is true that, by stretching these concepts sufficiently, a good deal can be brought in under this focusing umbrella -- including much that those with a different "gut feeling" on the issue would call rationalization or irrelevancy. At this stage, some people might want to debate questions about the nature of personhood, or even about the major premise's validity itself. Ethics, however, is partly a process of bracketing out potentially unresolvable issues in favor of reaching a conclusion.   Thus, it puts at least some limits on the sorts of normative thinking that can be brought in at this stage.

(2) A deductive syllogism is not the only form of application that we would classify under this model. At least some forms of utilitarian calculation share the characteristic features of this model of application, so they will be classified here as well.   In the act-utilitarian method, the entire normative force is contributed by the utilitarian principle: One ought to do the act which would produce the greatest good for the greatest number. No additional *normative* reasoning is employed in applying the principle to a particular situation. All that is done here is to predict the likely consequences of various alternatives for action (perhaps also calculating their probability) and to sum their positive and negative features.   The procedure of decision-making for an act-utilitarian can be characterized in terms of the following steps:

1) articulating all the alternatives for action in the situation which are in any way possible;

2) predicting the likely consequences of each alternative;

3) measuring these consequences in terms of selected quantitative (and perhaps also qualitative) parameters -- for purposes of illustration, let us consider a hedonistic utilitarian, who would measure only the parameters of pleasure and pain;

4) summing these measurements for each alternative in some way (e.g., Bentham's proposed "hedonic calculus");

5) comparing the balance of positive and negative measurements for each alternative ("the balance of good over evil"); and

6) selecting the alternative which produces the greatest balance of good over evil (e.g., pleasure over pain).

See figure 2 for a representation of this process.

None of these steps in themselves require normative reasoning. The process is wholly one of following logical rules such as prediction, classification, measurement, and even statistical probabilities. We call

Figure 2

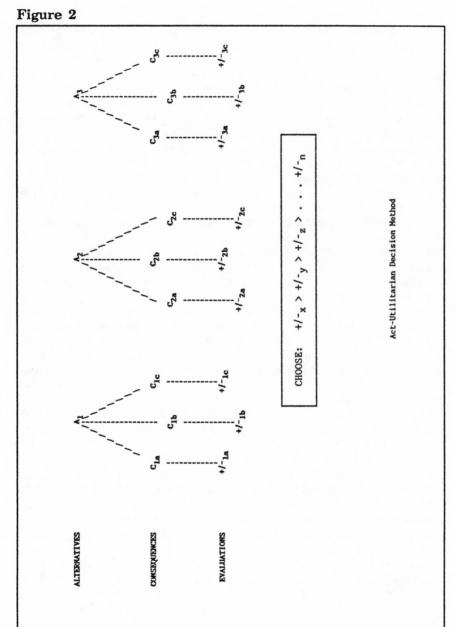

Act-Utilitarian Decision Method

these "rules" in the sense introduced in chapter 1. Inasmuch as there can be different causal theories to form the basis of prediction and different understandings of the theoretical calculus of probabilities, extrinsic or procedural interpretants are introduced. Note, however, that these are *not* normative elements. Indeed, one feature that most appealed to Bentham and Mill about the utilitarian method was precisely the possibility it permitted of resolving ethical problems through the methods of science. Thus it closely matches contemporary decision theory (of which it is the progenitor).

One could measure the amounts of pleasure and pain likely to result from the alternatives, sum these up, and compare the totals without having made any judgment that pleasure is good and ought to be chosen and that pain is bad and ought to be avoided. These normative judgments are *external* to the process of prediction and measurement, telling us what to do with the results of this process, but not directly shaping the process itself (except in the limited -- and not in itself normative -- way of directing our attention to one sort of consequence rather than another). It is left to the utilitarian principle of obligation and the hedonist theory of nonmoral value to supply the normative force of the argument.

Thus, one important source of the application model's attractiveness is that the normative aspects of reasoning and the descriptive aspects of calculation and measurement are neatly compartmentalized in different stages of the argument. The task of applied ethics, on this model, is *not* to justify the normative principle or to critically examine it, but rather simply to *apply* it to the situation at hand.

For an example of the application of this process, the board members who were evaluating Professor Jones's research protocol from an act-utilitarian perspective would try to predict as carefully as possible all the effects, both immediate and remote, of carrying out these specific procedures on the particular subjects likely to be chosen. This would involve judgments of probability and attempts to quantify consequences of various sorts (i.e., the intensity, duration, etc., of pleasures and pains likely to be involved), but none of these are inherently normative judgments. The normative force is contributed entirely by the utilitarian principle.

It might be useful to give another example of this sort of reasoning, if only because the notion of a research protocol (involving, as it does, a series of *rules* by which the experiment will be conducted) may be thought to be intrinsically incompatible with an act-utilitarian approach to moral decision-making. It is instructive to note, however, that the formulation of research in terms of a "principled" protocol is prompted, not by ethical considerations, but by the demands for consistency and controlled variation dictated by the canons of scientific rigor.

Nevertheless, whatever the implications of such an approach for the scientific rigor of the research, the ethical method of act-utilitarianism would dictate a presumption that Professor Jones should avoid conducting his project in terms of a rigid protocol, and instead should make decisions about whom to enlist in the project and how conduct it on a case-by-case or step-by-step basis. Then he would make these decisions by predicting the consequences of alternative actions open to him in each specific situation. For example, an oncologist acting under the act-utilitarian method of ethical analysis might conduct herself as follows: after an extensive work-up and evaluation of a patient, she might phone the statistician responsible for assigning random numbers and say: "Hey, Judy, give me a randomization in which my patient receives adriamycin. This lady really needs adriamycin." Thus, the oncologist is predicting (or has a gut feeling about) a negative outcome for her patient if the patient does not receive adriamycin.[*]

Here again, the normative force would enter only through the general utilitarian principle, and not in the course of the prediction and measuring of consequences.

(3) Proponents of this model of reasoning are likely to eschew attempts to develop a distinctive "biomedical ethics." In their view, general ethical principles can be applied directly to any context, including medicine, without need for intervening normative elements to guide application. Thus, for example, K. Danner Clouser[2] once insisted that bioethics is "the same old ethics" applied to problems in health care. His reason for making this point was to demonstrate the continuity between medical ethics and other aspects of ethical theory. Consider, for example, the following passage from his essay:

> "Do not kill" is a moral rule. It would not be this rule itself that would be challenged or justified within medical ethics. Nor would medical ethics as such be concerned with articulating and defending criteria for exceptions to the rule. Rather medical ethics prepares the ground for the constructions of ordinary ethics. Is withdrawing lifesaving therapy an instance of killing? Is the refusal to initiate a life-support system an instance of killing? Are we killing one when we give the limited lifesaving facilities to another instead? We are not questioning whether we should kill or not; we accept

---

[*] Of course, this approach is not permitted by the canons of scientific research. Double-blind studies rule out the investigator's bias. Yet pre-randomization by hunch does remain a problem. See *Journal of Medicine and Philosophy*, (1986). Edited by K. Schaffner.

that "ordinary" moral rule. What we are questioning is whether, in these special and difficult situations, our action is appropriately labeled "killing."[3]

(4) Richard McCormick's[4] response to the position of Paul Ramsey on pediatric research might also be construed as an example of application-model reasoning (although we will offer an alternative -- and, we believe, more accurate -- reading of McCormick's position in chapter 3). McCormick points towards a deductive model when he claims that what he is doing is "unpacking" the notion of parental consent. McCormick's argument might be characterized in terms of the set of practical syllogisms 2d, 2e, 2f (which should be contrasted with Ramsey's position, set out in syllogisms 2a through 2c above.)

(5) A third contributor to the debate regarding nontherapeutic research on children, William G. Bartholome,[5] also follows the application model -- but in a utilitarian form. His claim is that participation in nontherapeutic research (being an altruistic act, embodying regard for the welfare of others) can contribute to moral growth; and this is the basis for legitimate parental consent on behalf of their children. Their proxy consent is an expression of parental obligation to promote moral growth on the part of their children. This is best interpreted as a variety of utilitarian reasoning, in which moral development is seen as a (or perhaps the) fundamental intrinsic good.

(6) R. M. Hare[6] reveals an application-model stance when he criticizes past discussions of the issue of abortion (and, in particular, the well-known article by Judith Jarvis Thomson[7]) on the grounds that they do not derive their conclusions from a general ethical theory. His recent book[8] tries to establish that ethical conclusions can be adequately derived from a rule utilitarian theory. The assumption that all moral conclusions must be rooted in a deductive way in general principles or theory is an expression of application-model thinking. Hare's general doctrine of a "logic" of imperatives[9] can be seen as presupposing an application model as the only acceptable style of moral reasoning.

(7) We shall argue in chapter 3 that Robert Veatch's contractarian theory of medical ethics amounts, in the last analysis, to an instance of the mediation model. However, certain elements of his argument can be interpreted best as examples of the application model. For example, when he considers the issue of proxy consent for incompetent patients, Veatch speaks, not of creating exceptions to the principle of autonomy, but rather of what he describes as a proposal to "extend the concept of autonomy to familial autonomy."[10] He claims that the family constitutes a *moral community* and maintains: "Any full theory of medical ethics must include a theory of these moral communities."[11]

2d

Moral principle:	One ought to treat each person as an end-in-himself or herself and never merely as a means.
Descriptive Premise:	To use a person as a subject in nontherapeutic research without obtaining morally valid consent is to treat him or her merely as a means.
Conclusion:	One ought never to use a person as a subject in nontherapeutic research without obtaining morally valid consent.

2e

Normative premise:	One ought never to use a person as a subject in nontherapeutic research without obtaining morally valid consent.
Descriptive premise:	Parental consent on behalf of a child is morally valid "precisely insofar as it is a reasonable presumption of the child's wishes" and this judgment of the child's wishes, in turn, can be derived from judgments about what the child *ought* to have wanted.
Policy Conclusion:	One ought never to use a child as a subject in nontherapeutic research unless a) parental consent is obtained and b) this consent is based on valid judgments about what the child *ought* to wish.

2f

Normative premise:	One ought never to use a child as a subject in nontherapeutic research unless a) parental consent is obtained and b) this consent is based on valid judgments about what the child *ought* to wish.
Descriptive premise:	The research protocol that Professor Jones proposes to undertake comprises nontherapeutic research on young children, but their parents have consented to their participation based upon valid judgments about what the child *ought* to wish.
Practical Conclusion:	Professor Jones's protocol may be implemented.

In other words, rather than applying additional normative analysis to the principle of autonomy in order to work out exceptions to or modifications of it, he seeks to interpret the notion of the entity possessing autonomy in a way that will bring the actions of the family under this principle. *The normative force of the principle remains unaltered.* Its range of application is changed by means of conceptual moves which are not in themselves normative.

(8) A very similar maneuver is taken by James Rachels in his comments on a paper by R. M. Hare. Distinguishing between "being alive" (in the biological sense) and "having a life" (in what some have called "the biographical sense"), Rachels argues for an interpretation of the moral prohibition against killing which would incorporate only the latter sense:

> I don't think it is desirable for us to cling to a strict rule against killing if we understand the point of that rule to be the preservation of living things simply for the sake of preserving living things. It is desirable, however, that we cling to a rule protecting *lives*. In sketching the implications of such a rule, I think I have only been drawing out the implications of the rule we already have, but which we often   misunderstand.[12]

The last sentence of this quotation is quite revealing. It indicates rather obviously that Rachels sees himself working within the deductive application model.

(9) In an interesting exchange on the issue of monetary payments for participation in research,[13] Lisa Newton[14] approaches the issue from the application model when she hangs the entire debate from the peg of the principle of autonomy and its antipaternalistic implications. For this, she is taken to task by Ruth Macklin,[15] who points out that numerous principles are involved with this matter and a satisfactory resolution of the issue requires some attempt to weigh the force of all of them (in a process we shall classify under the mediation model in chapter 3), and find a balance between them. Newton has since argued together with a physician colleague that the principle of autonomy and the method of deductive application should be modified in light of a dialogue between physician and ethicists in the clinical setting.[16]

Macklin also illustrates another interesting example of the application model in the course of her response to Newton. The National Commission for the Protection of Human Subjects attempts a deductive-looking move when they interpret the principle of respect for persons to include what we would call paternalistic actions towardsincompetent patients (although Macklin herself would not so classify them). They put the point this way:

> Respect for persons incorporates at least two basic ethical
> convictions: First, that individuals should be treated as autonomous
> agents, and second, that persons with diminished autonomy are
> entitled to protection.[17]

This is obviously an attempt to "expand" the root principle
without challenging its normative force directly. Since this purports
to be a move in conceptual analysis -- i.e., a specification of the
meaning of "respect for persons" -- we classify it as a piece of
application-model reasoning. Critics of this maneuver may very well
argue that it incorporates covert normative reasoning -- i.e., smuggling
in an independent norm of protection or benevolence under the guise
of conceptual analysis. Indeed, as we shall see in the next chapter,
Ronald Dworkin maintains that *all* judicial-style reasoning actually
incorporates independent normative judgment. If either of these
claims turns out to be correct, the above example will have to be
reclassified as mediation-model reasoning. We shall examine these
claims in some detail in chapter 3.

(10) H. T. Engelhardt, Jr., in his *The Foundations of Bioethics*,
argues that autonomy is a condition of possibility of morality.[18]
Engelhardt claims that the primary moral and political responsibility
of a pluralistic society is to keep the peace. The best way to keep a
peaceable society is to respect individual autonomy and self-
determination as far as possible. Respecting autonomy makes
negotiations about values in relationships possible. In this way,
respect for an individual's values is guaranteed. Mutual respect
defines moral persons; lack of respect for persons characterizes
outlaws from morality.[19]

Traditionally, paternalism has been contrasted to autonomy. That
element of paternalism that seeks the good of the other person,
beneficence, is seen by Engelhardt as vacuous compared to the
primacy of autonomy in medical ethics. The reason for this is that
the interpretation of the good depends upon diverse cultural influences
as well as individual judgments. Early in his argument, Engelhardt
views autonomy as setting the boundaries of autonomy while
beneficence might define its content. Thus, autonomy conditions
morality; beneficence offers for one's consideration "what is good or
bad to do" in specific contexts as well as in general overarching
considerations. Clearly, this libertarian approach places the principle
of autonomy prior to the principle of beneficence. Freedom precedes
the good:

> Respect of the principle of autonomy binds all persons together in
> a moral life. Respect of particular principles of beneficence

separates communities.   Respect of the general principle of
beneficence reminds individuals from different moral communities
of the common commitment to doing the good, even when the
visions of the good diverge.[20]

Autonomy is then defined as a maxim: "Do not do to others that
which they would not have done to them, and do for them that which
one has contracted to do."[21]   In this view the role of beneficence is
subsumed under autonomy.   As the basis of a community's, a
profession's, or a person's articulation of values and beliefs, beneficence
gradually drops out of Engelhardt's analysis.   He pursues the
ascendancy of autonomy to its logical consequences.
     In fact, this approach is nothing new for Engelhardt.   In an
earlier work, the emphasis on autonomy led him to the acceptance of
its consequences, without much of a concomitant reflection on the
possibility of the inadequacy of the reasoning process itself. Of course,
such a self-critical move would depend upon one's hesitancy about the
morality of the conclusions towards which one's logic drives:

> One must be willing, as a price for recognizing the freedom of
> others, to live with the consequences of that freedom: some persons
> will make choices that they would regret were they to live longer.[22]

When autonomy becomes the first condition of morality, even
though the consequences of the primacy of autonomy are seen as
unfortunate, one must be willing to tolerate those actions with which
one disagrees and feels impelled by conscience to oppose.   Hence in
his book, Engelhardt argues for the rightness of the consequences of
his theory--infanticide, abortion, assisted suicide, and direct euthanasia,
all hallmarks of a libertarian moral agenda. His underlying argument
is represented in syllogism 2g.
     There are a number of objections to this thesis.[23] Despite them,
one must be willing to grant the persuasiveness of Engelhardt's point
of view.   To object appears to disvalue the importance of human
freedom.   In the end, however, it is easier to accept his view when
applied to dying patients, or to the self-determination of individuals
facing the enormous power of contemporary medicine, than it would
be to extrapolate it as a general ethical theory. Consider, for example,
the autonomous individual who infringes upon the rights of others.
Or consider the libertarian duty to tolerate other individuals' freedoms
that violate fundamental perceptions of human good. Does this mean
that, for example, the Nazi elimination of the retarded, socialists,
Jews, and gypsies, in spite of common human commitments to the
value of human life, must be tolerated? In these instances, at least,
the good seems to take precedence over autonomy.   Indeed, if one

---

2g

Major premise:	The primary moral and political responsibility of a pluralistic society is to keep the peace.
Minor premise:	The best way to keep a peaceable society is to respect individual autonomy and self-determination as far as possible.
Conclusion:	The primary moral and political responsibility of a pluralistic society is to respect individual autonomy and self-determination.

Maxim:	Do not do to others that which they would not have done to them, and do for them that which one has contracted to do.

---

autonomous entity's rights can check another's freedom, then autonomy itself cannot be the primary principle. Rather, as we have argued, there is no single primary principle, but a balance of fundamental ones.

If there is a fundamental principle, it must be so generally contentless, that it hardly counts as a fundamental principle. The condition of possibility of a moral life, for example, cannot be seen as freedom *per se*, but human freedom to "articulate, defend, and pursue the good."[24] Freedom does not stand naked, even for Kant and Mill. It is circumscribed by obligations. Freedom is in balance with the "ought." Even the original notion of rights contained an element of obligations: they were freedoms to do what one ought to do.[25]

(11) A convenient summary of the application mode of deductive reasoning can be extracted from Sally Gadow's effort to argue in favor of elderly patients' decision-making on the grounds that autonomy takes precedence over beneficence, or in her words, "at times, autonomous patient decisions defy medical definitions of benefit"[26] The logic of her argument is as shown in syllogism 2h and 2i.

The indicated course of action of this reasoning would require patient-centered health-care transactions in which the elderly would guide the physician. Some workable models of this idea are possible, despite the persistent and enduring evidence that the majority of patients do not want to guide their doctors about what would benefit them.

To recapitulate: this model of ethical reasoning places all the normative force in the major premise of the practical syllogism. Determining what to do in a particular situation of action requires only nonnormative reasoning to interpret the norm and apply it to the context at hand.

2h

Normative premise:	The purpose of medicine is to benefit patients.
Descriptive premise:	But benefit is best defined as a course of action that has the greatest possibility of facilitating or restoring autonomy.
Conclusion:	The purpose of medicine is to restore autonomy.

2i

Normative premise:	The purpose of medicine is to restore autonomy.
Descriptive premise:	But the notion of autonomy entails the notion that patients can best define their own benefits.
Policy conclusion:	The purpose of medicine is to help patients identify and define their own benefits, not to act on the basis of what doctors think they need.

B. Strengths of the Application Model

The application approach, bringing theory to bear on practice, has at least three strong points to recommend it.

First -- and what is undoubtedly a primary source of its appeal to philosophers -- its deductive style is neat and orderly and indicates rigor. The practical syllogisms into which we cast the arguments of Ramsey and McCormick represent an apogee of this achievement.

Lewis Carroll[27] taught us long ago that a rigorous form of argument does not end the possibility for disputes, although it may shift their locus.   In the same way, the attempt at rigorous formulation of arguments does have the considerable virtue of isolating the elements of the argument from one another and sorting out the different components stating the position. This can, indeed, be helpful in any critical examination of the debate, since it assists us in focusing attention on the aspects central to the controversy.

In the Ramsey-McCormick debate, for example, it is instructive to note that both of the disputants begin with the same fundamental ethical principle -- that is, the Kantian injunction that persons must never be treated *merely* as means. The dispute begins at the first step of interpretation of this form of the categorical imperative -- where Ramsey insists that there can be no substitute for individual informed and voluntary consent (according to him, anything else amounts to treating the subject merely as a means). McCormick, by contrast, accepts a wider category of "morally valid consent" which can be seen in the next stage of interpretation and application to include a carefully circumscribed parental consent. Thus the same principle has been conjoined with two different axioms of application.

The issue to consider, then, in critically examining this debate, is which of these interpretations is arguably the most accurate in capturing the meaning of the Kantian principle. On this point, we would contend that Ramsey wins the round. The root notion in the Kantian system is *autonomy*. To treat persons as *ends* is, fundamentally, to acknowledge and respect their autonomy. But it is nothing less than a contradiction in terms to speak (as McCormick's interpretation requires us to do) of a *proxy* exercising *autonomy* on someone else's behalf. This would amount to action that is both *self-directed* (autonomous) and directed *by another* (proxy) at the same time! (This criticism may be unfair to McCormick. As we shall see in chapter 3, the most plausible interpretation of his argument is not the application of Kant portrayed here.)

Incidentally, the Belmont Report's interpretation of the principle of respect for persons (quoted in example #9 above) is questionable in the same way. It would be more plausible to say (as, for example, the *Conroy*[28] court has done) that the principle of respect for autonomy is *no longer applicable* when the patient's autonomy is diminished, rather than to attempt to reinterpret the principle of respect for autonomy into a norm of *protection*.

However, this round does not complete the debate. Discussion may shift to another normative premise -- such as, for example, the claims brought into the debate by Bartholome.

A second strength of the application position is that (except possibly in its act-utilitarian form) it obviously and emphatically embodies "acting on principle." The normative thrust in this pattern of reasoning is wholly contributed by the moral principle which comprises the major premise of the practical syllogism; and it compels one to conclude that it is respect for this principle which motivates one to action when he or she makes a decision on the basis of such reasoning. Charles Fried, in his book *Right and Wrong*, gives an especially thorough and engaging account of the appeal of principles (and, indeed, absolute or unexceptionable principles) in moral decision-making and action:

> It is part of the idea that lying or murder are wrong, not just bad, that these things you must not do -- no matter what. They are not mere negatives that enter into a calculus to be outweighed by the good you might do or the greater harm you might avoid. Thus the norms which express deontological judgments -- for example, Do not

commit murder -- may be said to be absolute . . . . Even within
such boundaries we can imagine extreme cases where killing an
innocent person may save a whole nation. In such cases it seems
fanatical to maintain the absoluteness of the judgment, to do right
even if the heavens fall. And so the catastrophic may cause the
absoluteness of right and wrong to yield, but even then it would be
a non sequitur to argue (as consequentialists are fond of doing) that
this proves that judgments of right and wrong are always a matter
of degree, depending on the relative goods to be attained and harms
to be avoided. I believe, on the contrary, that the concept of the
catastrophic is a distinct concept just because it identifies the
extreme situations in which the usual categories of judgment
(including the category of right and wrong) no longer apply. At the
other end of the spectrum, there is the concept of the trivial, the
de minimis where the absolute categories do not yet apply.[29]

There is a strong tradition in ethical theory -- most prominently
identified with Kant, Prichard, and C. A. Campbell -- which holds that
action "on principle" is a *sine qua non* of genuinely *moral* action.
Other motivations are "heteronomous," to use Kant's term -- which
means that they are conditional upon motivations we happen to have,
and thus liable to be abandoned if our inclinations undergo alteration
(or our virtue lost). For example, a physician who spends a great
deal of time with his or her patients and shows deep concern for them
out of a feeling of benevolent affection may be a splendid physician,
indeed -- but then something might happen that may weaken or
destroy benevolent affection. Perhaps a patient will come along that
rubs the physician the wrong way, or perhaps events in his or her
personal life will lead "the mind of the philanthropist [to be] clouded
by sorrow of his own, extinguishing all sympathy with the lot of
others."[30] In this situation, the physician who was guided previously
by inclination is likely to cease the practices that we found admirable
and, instead, to become cold and indifferent towardspatients. But
"now suppose that he tears himself out of this dead insensibility, and
performs the action without any inclination to it, but simply from
duty, then first has his action its genuine moral worth."[31]
    This theory that only action on principle has moral worth or
value has a certain appeal to it. We shall be on the lookout, in the
chapters to follow, for alternative accounts of moral reasoning and
whether these can provide a theory of moral value which is equally
satisfactory.* We also shall consider criticisms of this account which
would be raised from the various perspectives we examine.

---

* See especially chapter 7 below, where we discuss alternative conceptions
of virtue.

A third strength of the application reasoning model is that it firmly counters ethical relativism by offering objective, generalizable normative standards on the basis of which any specific course of action can be criticized. As we shall see, this sharply contrasts both with forms of "situation ethics" and with virtue-theories, each of which seems liable to degenerate into person-relative norms and thus into a vague sort of relativism. It is certainly true that there can be disputes about the interpretation and application of principles. We saw a clear example of this in the exchange between Ramsey and McCormick on nontherapeutic research involving children. However, there can be no suggestion under this model that *both* interpretations might be correct, or that it might be a matter of individual taste or choice which of the two competing applications to make to a specific situation. If two theorists arrive at different situational applications of the same principle, then, on the application-model point of view, at least one of them must be mistaken; and the mistake can in principle be traced to an error of interpretation or deduction. It may be difficult to determine which one (if either) of them is correct, but there is no room for the suggestion that *both* might be.

C. Weaknesses of the Application Model
The criticism most often brought against the application model method is that it can degenerate into "legalism" -- that is, dedication to rules in and of themselves even when they do not serve any morally compelling purpose. Joseph Fletcher, Dietrich Bonhoeffer, and other "situation ethics" proponents have raised this point forcefully. For example, Fletcher says:

> With [the legalist] approach one enters into every decision-making situation encumbered with a whole apparatus of prefabricated rules and regulations. Not just the spirit but the letter of the law reigns. Its principles, codified in rules, are not merely guidelines or maxims to illuminate the situation; they are directives to be followed. Solutions are preset, and you can "look them up" in a book -- a Bible or a confessor's manual.[32]

A more clinically oriented expression of this same criticism can be seen in the call for an end to *all* "routine" procedures in a recent document entitled "Patients' Rights: A Five Point Agenda for the 80s." This document, which was distributed by George J. Annas at a 1981 National Conference on Patients' Rights, reads as follows:

> "NO 'ROUTINE' PROCEDURES." Procedures should be performed only if specifically indicated, not because they are 'routine' -- e.g., routine admissions tests, Johnnies, wheelchairs for in-hospital transport, sleeping pills, etc.[33]

The hospital policies specified here as the object of the charge of excessive legalism can hardly be said to have the status of fundamental moral principles. They are closer to the level of policies that we will discuss below in chapter 4 under the validation model. However, the spirit of this criticism applies equally well (or, perhaps, even more aptly) to application reasoning.

Consider, as another example, the physician who has determined in his or her own mind, through an application-model process of reasoning, that direct abortion is *never* morally justified in any situation for any reason. He or she might stand agonizingly by and allow both a pregnant woman and her baby to die in a situation in which the mother's life might have been saved through a direct abortion. His or her role-specific duties to save life will have been abandoned. Most critics of this physician's action would challenge the interpretation and/or deduction by which this position was reached; but, above and beyond that, they would also condemn the action as "rule worship" -- that is, allegiance to an abstract principle in preference to the immediate value of a human life.

This is also part of what is wrong with a bill recently passed by the Illinois legislature which, citing grounds of conscience, dictates that no physician who has moral objections to abortion need "perform, assist, counsel, suggest, recommend, refer, or participate in diagnostic testing to detect fetal abnormalities, which may lead to abortion . . . ."[34]

This is the dark side of "acting on principle," and it has been subject to sharp criticism since the days of Kant. Fried[35] attempts to side-step this criticism in his own application system (and he would undoubtedly claim that Kant is entitled to the same defense) by arguing that all his fundamental principles are themselves expressions of respect for persons. Thus, far from being abstract norms which compete with humanitarian goals, these principles express the deepest meaning of -- and provide an essential condition for -- the moral significance of humanitarian concern.

A related criticism of the application model is the claim that it lacks sensitivity to the context of decision. The example cited just above of the "principled" anti-abortionist also illustrates this point. The context is one that contains the important value of the mother's life, and yet this seems to be ignored in the process of deduction and interpretation. Consider another example. Examine the viewpoint of Dr. Emerson in the drama "Whose Life Is It Anyway?" His single-minded dedication to preserving the life of his patients blinds him to the values of Ken Harrison, the quadriplegic sculptor, and his rationally-arrived-at decision to forego further treatment.

This may be a valid criticism of a form of application reasoning which regards only certain limited features of the context of action as morally relevant; but it may well be that it is more often a matter of deficient thoroughness in the process of application rather than a failure of the application model as such. In most comprehensive ethical systems all of the features of the situation which we would consider pre-analytically to be morally relevant do, in fact, link up with one or more of the principles.

Thus, for example, the same principle or system from which the anti-abortion physician derives a rule prohibiting direct abortions may contain one or more principles from which one could derive a duty to preserve the mother's life -- that is, a principle of preserving life (such as that cited by Dr. Emerson in "Whose Life Is It Anyway?") or an interpretation of the Kantian principle which prohibits using any person (in this case, the mother) merely as a means, that is, as a means to upholding the doctor's very reasoning process. Thus, by taking respect for persons into account, the physician would, at the very least, be faced with a conflict of duties -- a duty, derived from one principle, which prohibits taking a baby's life; and another duty, derived from another equally fundamental principle, which dictates action to save the mother's life. Some mechanism (perhaps by means of reinterpretation of one or another aspect of the situation, in the spirit of deductive reasoning, or perhaps through mediation reasoning) would have to be used in order to attempt to resolve the conflict -- but, at least, this morally important feature of the situation would have been taken into account. In a parallel way, Dr. Emerson's allegiance to the principle of preserving life conflicts with acknowledgement of the patient's *rights* -- including the right to refuse treatment. Weighting of fundamental moral principles is a difficult task, however, for application reasoning.

It is possible that, even after Dr. Emerson and the anti-abortion physician have taken into account these morally relevant features of the situation, and have resolved the resulting conflicts of principle by some as yet unexplained mechanism, their position will remain unchanged. That is, it is possible that Dr. Emerson will conclude that preserving the life of his patient is the most important moral concern. Similarly, it is possible that the anti-abortion physician will conclude that avoiding direct killing must be his dominant moral concern. If this happens, the critics are unlikely to be pleased with the outcome. And they are likely to continue to challenge these moral conclusions. They are certainly entitled to do so. However, they can no longer challenge them *on the grounds that* they ignore elements of the context.

What we are emphasizing here is this: often a normative disagreement is portrayed as a procedural one. A person is accused of a procedural error (such as failing to take into account elements of the context) because he did not take them into account *in the right way* -- that is, he did not give the same weight to them that the critic would have given. But to put the matter in procedural terms is to mislocate the point of dispute. It ought to be discussed for what it is, a directly normative disagreement. Put another way, it is a disagreement about what weights are to be given conflicting fundamental moral principles in difficult contexts.

We conclude, then, that the legalism criticism is not as easily lodged against the application model as might initially be thought. A full-bodied application model *can* acknowledge the moral relevance of all plausible features of the context. However, it may still be regarded as a procedural defect in an ethical theory if the scope of this relevance is so opaque that it is frequently unnoticed by the average person who attempts to apply it as a guide to moral choice, or -- and this is more important -- ultimately so irrelevant in assisting interpreting principles that it can make no difference in the conclusion.

The application model is also criticized as failing properly to respect cultural and religious differences we might regard, pre-analytically, as morally relevant. Can an absolute injunction against suicide and other life-endangering actions, for example, be reconciled with respect for the Jehovah's Witnesses' deep religious qualms about accepting blood transfusions? Or, can the set of principles drawn from Western morality be validly applied to other cultures, which may have significantly different conceptions of health and illness, personal responsibility, and so on?

Finally, some take it as a defect of this model that agreement on fundamental principles does not assuredly lead to agreement on conclusions. This objection applies to Beauchamp and Childress's book on the principles of biomedical ethics. The neatness, orderliness, and rigor of the system would be expected to minimize the possibilities of moral disagreement. However, application-model reasoning still leaves plenty of room for dispute about the interpretation of features of the situation. There are at least three disputed arenas we have distinguished: (1) whether another general standard should be employed under which cases are to be considered; (2) the matter of how the general principle is to be interpreted in application to the situation at hand (as we saw above in the dispute between Ramsey and McCormick on nontherapeutic research involving children; this point includes disputes about axioms and rules, and internal and external interpretations of the principles); and (3) the question of how many of the general principles of the system are relevant to the situation at hand (as we saw above in the examples of Dr. Emerson and the anti-abortion physician).

When more than one general principle is brought into play, there is, of course, the possibility of conflicting directives for action. This is the moral quandary for Dr. Emerson and the anti-abortion physician.

Indeed, it is possible that a single principle could yield conflicting directives in a given situation.   For example, Kant's principle prohibiting treating any person merely as a means might be interpreted to direct *both* that action be taken to save the mother's life (lest *she* be treated as a means to service of some abstract principle) *and* that the baby not be directly killed (lest she or he be treated as a means to save the mother's life).   These possibilities of conflict, then, give rise to still a fourth source of dispute.   There may be different judgments about which of the conflicting directives should be given priority.

It is entirely possible that such disputes will in the last analysis prove intractable, indicating a serious limitation in the usefulness of the application approach in reaching concrete decisions in medical ethics.   The chief means of reconciling apparent conflicts which is open to the application model is to reexamine the principles involved and the (nonnormative) rules for interpretation of the situation which establishes the tie between the principle and the case at hand.   This is done in hopes that at least one of the conflicting directives will be seen not to follow from the fundamental principles after all, and thus, a course of action can be taken which will not violate "acting on principle."   As Fried says:

> absoluteness is only a suggestive first approximation of a much more complex characteristic. . . .   In every case the norm has boundaries and what lies outside those boundaries is not forbidden at all.   Thus lying is wrong, while withholding a truth which another needs may be perfectly permissible -- but that is because withholding truth is not lying.   Murder is wrong but killing in self-defense is not.   The absoluteness of the norm is preserved in these cases, but only by virtue of a process which defines its boundaries.   That process is different from the process by which good and bad are weighed in consequentialism, and so the distinctiveness of judgments of right and wrong is preserved.[36]

However, if reconciliation of conflicting directives should fail, it is unclear that application patterns of reasoning offer resources to resolve the conflict.   Any attempt to make a normative judgment about the relative weight of the conflicting principles would be a slide to mediation reasoning.   We will now examine that approach.

NOTES

1. Paul Ramsey, *The Patient as Person* (New Haven: Yale University Press, 1970), pp. 1-58. See also Paul Ramsey, "Some Rejoinders," *The Journal of Religious Ethics* 4, no. 2 (Fall 1976), pp. 185-237.

2. K. Danner Clouser, "Bioethics," *The Encyclopedia of Bioethics*, ed. Warren T. Reich (New York: Macmillan and Free Press, 1978), pp. 115-127.

3. Ibid., p. 117.

4. Richard McCormick, S.J.: "Proxy Consent in the Experimentation Situation," *Perspectives in Biology and Medicine* 18 (Autumn 1974), 2-20; "Experimentation in Children: Sharing in Sociality," *Hastings Center Report* 6 (December 1976), 41-46.

5. William G. Bartholome: "The Ethics of Nontherapeutic Research on Children," *Appendix to Report and Recommendation -- Research Involving Children*, The National Commission for the Protection of Human Subjects of Biomedical and Behavioral Research. (Washington, DC: U. S. Government Printing Office, 1977), DHEW Publication no. (OS) 77-00005, see especially pp. 3-17.

6. R. M. Hare, "Abortion and the Golden Rule," *Philosophy and Public Affairs* 4 (Spring 1975), 201-222.

7. Judith Jarvis Thomson, "A Defense of Abortion," *Philosophy and Public Affairs* 1 (Fall 1971), 47-66.

8. R. M. Hare, *Moral Thinking: Its Levels, Methods, and Point* (Oxford: Oxford University Press, 1981).

9. Cf. *Language of Morals*, pp. 17-55.

10. Robert M. Veatch, *A Theory of Medical Ethics* (New York: Basic Books, 1981), p. 213.

11. Ibid., p. 209.

12. James Rachels, "Comments on Professor Hare's Paper," *Philosophical Medical Ethics: Its Nature and Significance*, ed. Stuart F. Spicker and H. Tristram Engelhardt, Jr. (Boston: D. Reidel, 1977), pp. 68-69.

13. Ruth Macklin, "On Paying Money to Research Subjects," *IRB: A Review of Human Subjects Research* 3, no. 5 (May 1981), 1-6.

14. Lisa H. Newton, "Inducement, Due and Otherwise," *IRB: A Review of Human Subjects Research* 4, no. 3 (March 1982), 4-6.

15. Ruth Macklin, "Response: Beyond Paternalism," *IRB: A Review of Human Subjects Research* 4, no. 3 (March 1982), 6-7.

16. David G. Smith and Lisa H. Newton, "Physician and Patient: Respect for Mutuality," *Theoretical Medicine* 5, no. 1 (February 1984), 43-60.

17. National Commission for the Protection of Human Subjects of Biomedical and Behavioral Research, *The Belmont Report*, p. 4 (quoted in Macklin, "Response," p. 6).

18. H. Tristram Engelhardt, Jr., *The Foundations of Bioethics* (New York: Oxford University Press, 1986).

19. Ibid. p. 80.

20. Ibid., p.84.

21. Ibid., p. 86.

22. *Bartling v. Superior Court*, 209 Cal. Reptr. 70 (1984); *Bartling v. Glendale Adventist Medical Center*, 229 Cal. Reptr. 360 (1986).

23. As contrasts to his view of the nature of autonomy see, for example, Robert Veatch, "Autonomy's Temporary Triumph," *Hastings Center Report* 14 (October 1984), 38-40; Daniel Callahan, "Autonomy: A Moral Good, Not a Moral Obsession," *Hastings Center Report* 14 (October 1984), 41; Robert Morison, "The Biological Limits on Autonomy," *Hastings Center Report* 14 (October, 1984); David Jackson and Stuart Youngner, "Patient Autonomy and 'Death with Dignity,'" *New England Journal of Medicine* 301 (1979), 404-408. See also Edmund D. Pellegrino and David C. Thomasma, *For the Patient's Good: The Restoration of Beneficence in Health Care* (New York: Oxford University Press, 1988), pp. 44-50.

24. Pellegrino and Thomasma, *For the Patient's Good*, pp. 37-51.

25. Center for the Study of Democratic Institutions Staff, *Natural Law and Modern Society* (Salem, NH: Ayer Co., facsimile reproduction of the 1963 edition).

26. Sally Gadow, "Medicine, Ethics, and the Elderly," *The Gerontologist* 20 (1980), 680-685.

27. Lewis Carroll, "What the Tortoise Said to Achilles," *Mind* 4, no. 14 (April 1895), 278-280.

28. *Conroy, Matter of Claire*, 190 NJ Super 453, 464 A2d 303 (NJ App 1983) appeal docketed, No. 21, 642 (NJ Sup Ct); 98 N.J. 321, 486 A2d 1209 (1985).

29. Charles Fried, *Right and Wrong* (Cambridge, MA: Harvard University Press, 1978), pp. 9-10.

30. Immanuel Kant, *Foundations of the Metaphysics of Morals*, trans. by Lewis White Beck. Library of Liberal Arts. (Indianapolis: Bobbs-Merrill, 1959).

31. Ibid., p. 14.

32. Joseph Fletcher, *Situation Ethics* (Philadelphia: The Westminster Press, 1966), p. 18.

33. George Annas, unpublished paper, The National Conference on Patients' Rights, Nashville, TN, September 29-30, 1980.

34. Illinois House Bill 1415, as cited in an editorial by John C. Roberts and Donald H. J. Hermann in the *Chicago Tribune* (9 August 1987), Section 4, 2.

35. Fried, *Right and Wrong*, pp. 28-29.

36. Ibid., p. 10.

CHAPTER THREE
The Mediation Model

The second model of the relation of theory to practice in medical ethics is one in which theory is *mediated*, in its application to practice, by one or more types of intervening normative thinking. The normative thrust of the "major premise" or fundamental ethical principle is supplemented by intermediate reasoning (axioms) of a normative sort.

This can be achieved in at least three ways: (a) by bringing in priority judgments to arbitrate conflicts between fundamental principles, (b) by giving normatively laden definitions for terms other than deontic operators, and (c) by developing normative interpretations to specify indeterminacies in fundamental principles.

The first two of these moves are illustrated in the following passage:

Suppose Nazi soldiers investigating a hospital in Germany in the late 1930s had asked the administrator whether there were any Jewish patients in the hospital. If the administrator insisted that the hospital had no Jewish patients, although he knew there were in fact several, how should we describe this exchange and, in particular, the administrator's statement? Consider two possibilities: (1) The administrator's statement is a *lie*, but the lie is justified because it is intended to save the lives of innocent patients. (2) The administrator's statement is not a lie, because his questioners have no right to the truth. In (1) "lying" may be defined as intentionally telling a person what one believes to be untrue in order to deceive him or her. In (2) "lying" may be defined as not giving the truth to a person to whom it is due. The first involves a "neutral and relatively definite description" of lying, while the second involves a "nonneutral and relatively indefinite description."[*] The first definition indicates what counts as lying or truthtelling, but not how much moral weight lying or truthtelling has. The second definition, however, indicates how much lying or truthtelling counts, but not what is to count as lying or truthtelling. Although the second approach holds that lying is always wrong, it leaves open

---

[*] Donald Evans, "Paul Ramsey on Exceptionless Moral Rules," *American Journal of Jurisprudence* 16(1971):184-214. See also Sissela Bok, *Lying: Moral Choice in Public and Private Life* (New York: Pantheon Books, 1978), pp. 13-16.

the question when the truth is *due* someone. The first approach could stress that the moral life often involves doing the "lesser of two evils." It may sometimes be necessary to lie in order to prevent a worse evil. Proponents of the second approach may stress the harmony rather than the conflict among various principles and rules once we appreciate their meaning and thus their range of applicability.[1]

Both of these approaches to resolving conflicts between principles involve the sort of reasoning we are calling "mediation" model thinking. In both cases, independent normative judgments -- above and beyond the normative thrust contributed by the initial normative premise -- are inserted into the reasoning process.

A. Priority Judgments

In the hospital administrator's first possibility, this added normative judgment is a judgment of priority between two conclusions reached by appeal to two moral principles. The reasoning here might be represented as shown in 3a.

The new normative element is the premise labeled "normative priority rule." It is clear that it involves an independent moral assessment of conflicting duties, going beyond anything that can be deduced from the two fundamental moral principles with which the argument began. This is an issue of "moral weight" (as Beauchamp and Childress indicate is the case in this example). Moral weight is something tacked on to the final judgment externally. Thus, in our terms, it is a "rule." Reasoning like this falls under the mediation model, in which conclusions are derived from principles but mediated through external moral considerations.

B. Definitional Mediation

In the other approach, the mediation occurs in the *definition* of a "lie." To incorporate a normative element into the definition of the term "lie" is to mediate the normative thrust of the "ought" in the moral principle "We ought not to lie" by a substantive interpretation (axiom) which introduces novel normative force. This contrasts with approaches (classified in the previous chapter as examples of application-model reasoning) which determine the application of a principle through a descriptive analysis of the concept. The reasoning here might be represented as shown in 3b.

Contrast the foregoing definition of a lie, for example, to Charles Fried's normatively neutral definition:

> lying is wrong, while withholding a truth which another needs may be perfectly permissible -- but that is because withholding truth is not lying.[2]

3a

Moral principle:	A hospital administrator has a duty to save the lives of innocent patients.
Factual premise:	For me to reveal the presence of these Jewish patients would be to fail to save their lives.
Conclusion:	I ought *not* to reveal their presence.

Moral principle:	Lying is wrong.
Factual premise:	To insist there are no Jewish patients in this hospital is a lie.
Conclusion:	I ought *not* to insist there are no Jewish patients in this hospital.

Conclusion 1:	I ought not to reveal their presence (else I will fail to save their lives).
Conclusion 2:	I ought *not* to insist there are no Jewish patients in this hospital (else I will be telling a lie).
Normative priority rule:	In this situation, saving lives is a *more pressing* duty than refraining from lying.
Conclusion:	I ought not to reveal their presence, even if this requires me to insist there are no Jewish patients in this hospital.

3b

Moral principle:	Lying is wrong.
Factual premise:	To insist there are no Jewish patients in this hospital is an untruth; but it is not a lie to say this to the Nazi soldiers, since they are not *due* the truth.
Conclusion:	It would *not be wrong* to insist there are no Jewish patients in this hospital.

For Fried, the normative thrust is entirely in the moral operator "wrong." No *additional* normative dimension is added by the definition of lying. Although the definition is crucial to the correct application of the moral principle, it is obtained through its descriptive elements rather than by means of any added normative element. Fried's analysis of the situation of the hospital administrator would have to take a different tack, perhaps dealing with it as shown in 3c.

3c

Conclusion 1:   I ought not to reveal the presence of Jewish patients in my hospital (else I will fail to save their lives).

Conclusion 2:   I ought not to insist there are no Jewish patients in this hospital (else I will be telling a lie).

Strategic principle: Perhaps I could avoid revealing the information without telling a lie by some evasive stratagem (although this risks some danger of harm to myself).

Conclusion: I ought to attempt the evasive stratagem.

This strategic principle is not a matter of deciding what to do by drawing entailments from a normative principle (and thus it is not, strictly speaking, *moral* reasoning). Rather, it is a matter of devising a course of action which does not *violate* any normative principles (and thus, by avoiding evil, *does* turn out to be a feature of moral conduct). Essentially, however, this is technical reasoning, rather than moral or ethical. The entire normative thrust is contributed by the (absolute) principles with which the analysis of the situation began.

Another example of the definitional form of the mediation model is found in Mary Anne Warren's[3] essay on abortion. She distinguishes between two senses of "human": "human in the genetic sense" (which has no implications for the possession of rights like a right to life) and "human in the moral sense" (which is equivalent to "is a full-fledged member of the moral community" and thus does imply the possession of rights, including the right to life). Michael Tooley makes a parallel move with the definition of "person."[4] In both these cases, the normative question of a duty to protect the fetus is modified by the application of the definition offered. It is argued that there is no duty to protect the life of a human (in the genetic sense); and, although there is a duty to protect the life of persons (for Warren, humans in the moral sense), it is questionable whether the fetus qualifies. A debate about classification of the fetus is thus made to intervene in attempts to apply the principle prohibiting killing to abortion.

C. Other Examples of Mediating Priority Judgments

(1) Sir David Ross's system of prima facie duties[5] also amounts to mediation-model reasoning. Application of the general principles of prima facie duty to specific situations proceeds in deductive fashion until a conflict of duties arises (as it almost invariably does). At that point, appeal is made directly to moral intuition (an extra deductive element) to determine which of the conflicting principles or sets of principles ought to take priority in the situation at hand. The process would proceed much like that illustrated in Example 3a above, except that the "normative priority rule" (which is the mediating element) would stem from moral intuition.

(2) A Rossian approach is illustrated in medical ethics in a discussion of terminating treatment written by one of the present authors together with two physicians.[6] Fifty distinct considerations are cited which are sometimes invoked on one side or the other of decisions to terminate life-sustaining treatment. Then these are applied to a sample case to show how they bear on specific decisions. In this case (as, it is maintained, will occur in most such cases), considerations both pro and con can be adduced and thus it is essential to determine which set of considerations possess most weight in the situation. We attempt to establish a set of priority principles for emergency situations,[7] but these are guidelines only and they are subject to reordering in the nonemergency situation.

(3) Another example of the priority-judgment form of the mediation model is found in Jonsen, Siegler, and Winslade's *Clinical Ethics*. Their view of the origin of applicable normative principles does not fit the patterns discussed so far. It will be discussed below in chapter 6, along with other views in which the ethical judgment "follows from a perception of the various facts, opinions, and circumstances."[8] However, whatever the *source* of these principles, they still recognize the possibility that these may conflict in concrete situations; and, in these circumstances, additional normative judgments -- external to the prior normative principles in terms of which the situation was initially analyzed -- must be brought in to determine priorities. This element of their position is clear in the following quotation:

> Assessing the importance of facts, opinions, and circumstances in the light of ethical categories is, of course, the most perplexing task. When facts, opinions, and circumstances are meshed with* our

---

* We shall examine this notion of being "meshed with" a moral principle in chapter 6.

ethical categories, we call them considerations. No ethical scales exist into which considerations can be poured until "importance" shows up on a precisely calibrated gauge. Still, rough measures can be made and are made in everyday life. In this book, the rough measures are established by setting the four categories in order of priority. . . . Our initial ranking of the order of ethical importance is (1) Patient Preference, (2) Medical Indications, (3) Quality of Life, (4) External Factors.[9]

This mechanism of introducing external principles of priority is quite common. One suspects that it is viewed as a way of preserving as much of the rigor of a deductive system as possible, while making the minimal compromise with a unitary deductive system which will enable one to deal with the recurrent problem of conflicts between principles. Mechanisms more in the spirit of a deductive system -- such as Fried's technique of close analysis of the descriptive meaning of the key concepts and the doctrine (rule) of the double effect -- yield conclusions that many have found unpalatable. Further, like all human tools, they have been subject to distortion in some hands and used as a basis for rationalization of past judgments originally held on other grounds rather than rational analysis or decision-making. But, by bringing in an external priority principle, grounds can be given for abridging one or the other principle in situations of conflict without abandoning a deductive-based system or a strong role for general principles altogether.

(4) Another example of the use of external priority judgments is seen in Beauchamp and McCullough's *Medical Ethics*. They begin their analysis of moral issues in medicine by setting out two models ("principles," in our terms) which operate in connection with these decisions: "beneficence," which they see as the exclusive focus of medical reasoning; and "autonomy," which they ascribe to the patient. They insist that conflict between these two principles is inevitable and frequent -- a point which they illustrate by analysis of certain cases. Then they comment on ways in which this conflict can be reconciled:

> The conflict generated by the two models [i.e., beneficence and autonomy] is an inescapable dimension of medical practice: a conflict between the patient's best interests understood from the perspective of medicine and the patient's best interests understood from the perspective of the patient. . . .
> The upshot is that the obligations generated by these models are all prima facie . . . . all moral principles seem noble and inviolable when stated free of conflict with other principles. But controversial problems for medical ethics arise when their applicability in circumstances of conflict must be determined. A central task of medical ethics is thus to fix the limits of each of the two models in light of the demands of the other. Because both

perspectives merit consideration, discretion is required in clinical decision-making.[10]

This is nicely illustrated in their discussion of truth telling, where they set out three guidelines for management of information which attempt to strike a balance between beneficence and autonomy.[11]

(5) Richard McCormick's[12] position on involving young children as subjects in nontherapeutic research can also be seen to follow the mediation-model approach. Rather than merely applying the principle of informed consent in a formalistic way (as Ramsey does, in our application-model examples set out in the preceding chapter), McCormick tinctures it with doctrines of charity and brotherhood/sisterhood, with the resulting conclusion that children have obligations towardssociety that would support enlisting them in nontherapeutic research even if they cannot themselves give free and informed consent to such procedures.

This interpretation is more in line with his general natural law approach (sketched in chapter 1 above) than the interpretation offered in chapter 2. Thus, we view this as the more accurate reading of McCormick's position.

(6) In some authors, the mediation of external principles is brought in only in specific contexts -- for example, in connection with issues of public policy. This version of mediation-model reasoning is illustrated in James Rachels's carefully structured analysis of the issue of euthanasia.[13] After responding to numerous key general objections to active euthanasia, he sums up the case *for* euthanasia in specific situations in the argument shown in 3d, a piece of application-model reasoning with a heavily utilitarian flavor.[14]

3d

1. If an action promotes the best interests of everyone concerned, and violates no one's rights, then that action is morally acceptable.

2. In at least some cases, active euthanasia promotes the best interests of everyone concerned and violates no one's rights.

3. Therefore, in at least some cases active euthanasia is morally acceptable.

When it comes to the issue of public policy about these matters, however, Rachels does not rely on this reasoning alone. Instead, he brings in an external principle to provide an added normative thrust which he deems needed to convert a situational conclusion into a matter of law and public policy:

> However, none of this really proves that active euthanasia ought to be legalized. We need to turn now to arguments that are addressed more directly to the issue of legalization. One such argument is the "argument from the right to liberty." According to this argument, each dying patient should be free to choose euthanasia, or to reject it, simply as a matter of personal liberty. No one, including the government, has the right to tell another what choice to make. If a dying patient wants euthanasia, that is a private affair; after all, the life belongs to the individual, and so that individual should be the one to decide.[15]

This, then, brings in a principle about the right to liberty of the individual which did not appear in the argument for active euthanasia in the specific case. That argument hinged on *interests* of the individual and nonimpingement on the rights of *others*. By introducing this principle at this point, public policy is made. Such policy is therefore not a direct application of moral reasoning, but rather a matter of "second order" reasoning in which additional normative considerations are dominant. (We will discuss other examples of policy formation in the next chapter.)

D. Mediating Specifications

(1) A third form of mediation-model reasoning is found in rule-utilitarianism. As we explained in chapter 2, act-utilitarianism embodies application-model reasoning -- a linear application of the utilitarian principle of comparative evaluation of consequences to the nonnormative features of the situation at hand. In contrast, rule-utilitarianism introduces mediation through rules or policies which, although themselves justified by utilitarian comparative evaluation, *replace* the utilitarian principle in concrete decision-making. Thus these rules become normative elements, distinct from the fundamental principle, which enter into reasoning about specific cases.

One of the clearest accounts of the logic of rule-utilitarian reasoning is found in Rawls's explanation[16] of the "practice" conception of rules and the distinction between justifying acts falling under a practice (which is done by reference to rules of the practice itself and not to the principle of utility) and justifying the practice (which is done by appeal to the utilitarian principle).

Furthermore, the claim that decisions should be based on rules, policies, or practices rather than on act-utilitarian direct application of the utilitarian principle is itself often supported by appeal to utilitarian considerations.   The primary   arguments in favor of a rule- or policy-based approach are those which appeal to efficiency and consistency. As regards efficiency, to take the trouble to calculate *all* possible effects on *all* members of the moral reference group afresh for *each* such decision would take enormous amounts of time. It would be a great time-saver to work through this sort of calculation once for each class of situations and henceforth act on the policy arrived at as a result of this calculation.   Even more serious than the time consumed by a thoroughgoing act-approach is the danger that some relevant factor will be overlooked on some occasions -- which might make a significant difference to the decision.

Consistency, by contrast, is not only a canon of reason but also a moral virtue. If a doctor were to refuse the parents' request for antibiotics today when the child's condition appeared to be a viral infection, and yet give another set of parents a prescription tomorrow in circumstances which were virtually identical, she could properly be charged with inconsistency, incompetency, or "unfairness." (Think of a child's reaction to such a perceived inconsistency in the actions of a parent, and you will see the moral relevance of this notion: "But you said yes to Johnny when he asked *the very same thing* yesterday! You like him best!"   In general, children are very sensitive to moral principles -- especially those which serve their own interests.)

(2) A good example of a formalist, or legalist, approach to the resolution of moral dilemmas from a deductive standpoint is provided by the Vatican's instruction on reproductive technologies.[17]   While important concerns about manipulating inchoate and therefore helpless forms of human life are raised by the document, its deductive reasoning from principles not widely established means that it is open to the charge of being unpersuasive.[18]

3e	
Major Premise:	Technology must always serve the good of human life (as embodied in the natural law), and not vice versa.
Minor Premise:	But reproductive technology often subjects human life to its own goals.
Normative Conclusion:	Reproductive technology that does not serve human life is morally prohibited.

The minor is defended using several explications. One is the notion that human life should not be objectified and manipulated. Thus, selling fetal brain tissue from aborted fetuses for research purposes would be a form of objectifying human life and using it to benefit others. This would be morally repulsive, according to the Vatican document's reasoning. But that example is more clearly questionable than using reproductive technology, such as *in vitro* fertilization (IVF) to aid childless couples. Here the document regards any manipulation of gametes as objectification prohibited by the natural law. The latter is now interpreted to include the natural forms of reproduction between husband and wife, even the natural rhythm of the bodies in the act of copulation, a rhythm that IVF clearly bypasses. This additional consideration is called the "inseparability principle." In the past the inseparability of unitive and procreative functions in the marital act prompted the Vatican to reject artificial means of birth control as well. Thus, ruled out would be any manipulation of sperm and egg outside of the womb, even if done with the husband's sperm and wife's egg, as well as the more morally difficult problems of donor sperm and egg, surrogate motherhood, and the like.

The entire document, proceeding as it does from moral principle to clear prohibitions, reads like a catalogue of dos and don'ts. As noted, the problem with such an approach as the basis of moral policy conclusions is that the premises are open to challenge, as well as the interpretations of the meaning of the premises. In this instance, is it true that technology (a human creative process) must always serve moral human ends? Might it not sometimes be morally neutral?[19] Can the inseparability principle be maintained as an interpretation of the natural law? It is often regarded as a very questionable extrapolation, a kind of physicalism that neglects personal relationships.[20] Can a procedure, like IVF, deprived of the "proper perfections" of the natural procreative act, be always judged wrong, just because it is, in McCormick's words, "second best"? Does the anti-objectification interpretation of the value of human life stand up to ethical scrutiny? It is clearly not always wrong to subject the body to the objective manipulation of medical science, for example, in surgery, especially if the end of the act is to bring about a moral good such as health, or in the case of IVF, a child.

In any case, the reasoning process is deductive, but defense of the minor premise takes the form of additional "principles" from the tradition of natural law theory. These normative or axiomatic statements are used to further concretize the meaning of the major premise. The human-life-precedes-technology principle is focused on the procreative question through the axioms. It is interpreted as applying to procreative questions through the axioms. The difficulty lies, not only in the generality of the principle (it may not always apply), but in the very conservative interpretation the document gives to the axioms as well.

(3)   Addressing "A Problem of Application," William Frankena offers a proposal which introduces similar mediation-model reasoning:

> Perhaps, then, one can argue that we need things like custom and law to help us to channel our activities in the way of applying the principles of beneficence and equality -- that society must provide us with a set of mores and institutions in terms of which to operate.[21]

With characteristic clarity and forthrightness, Frankena acknowledges (a) that these mores and institutions are themselves normative; (b) that they originate, not directly in the fundamental moral principles of beneficence and equality, but rather in corporate decisions of the society; and (c) that they shape the application of fundamental moral principles (as he puts it, they "help us to channel our activities in the way of applying" the principles).

For example, the principles of beneficence and equality may tell us that the life needs and developmental needs of children ought to be met; but they do not, in themselves, tell us who ought to contribute to meet the needs of this particular child, nor do they tell me which child's needs I ought to contribute to meeting. These duties are "imperfect obligations" which dictate action of a general type but do not specify determinately how the duty is to be carried out. However, when this imperfect obligation is coupled with an established social institution of the family, a specific and stringent "perfect obligation" results: I have a duty to provide for *my own child's* needs; and each child can rightfully expect to have his or her needs met *by members of her or his family*.

Other systems of institutions are possible (e.g., the extended families portrayed in Plato's *Republic*, the Israeli kibbutz, etc.), and, in a society which has one of these systems, our specific duties would be different than they are in our society with our fabric of institutions. Thus, the normative content of the institutions serves to mediate the fundamental principles in application to the specific case.

An example in the area of medical ethics is given in 3f.

(4) Bernard Gert's system of moral rules[22] is at core a form of negative rule-utilitarianism. (Note that his definition of rules is different from our own.) The ten fundamental moral rules are established on a basis (the public moral attitude of rational persons) which amounts largely (although not totally) to a matter of minimizing negative consequences. Gert acknowledges this when he says, "the moral rules might be summarized as 'Don't cause evil' or 'Don't do that which will or is likely to cause anyone to suffer evil.'"[23] A part

3f

Principle of utilitarianism:	One ought to promote benefit and prevent harm.
Descriptive premise:	One way to promote benefit and prevent harm is to provide for this person's pressing health needs.
Conclusion:	Someone or other ought to provide for this person's pressing health needs. (Imperfect obligation.)
Institutional premise:	I am this person's physician (having established a relationship with him in the past on the basis of a mutual agreement between us).
Conclusion:	I ought to provide for this person's pressing health needs. (Perfect Obligation.)

of what is meant by calling it a moral rule is the attitude that violations are wrong and should be punished.

But his system also includes an account of "when it is morally justifiable to violate the rules" and this introduces separate normative (and even virtue) considerations. On his view, violation would be morally justified "only when one would publicly advocate such a violation."

> the considerations that are relevant to deciding whether to publicly advocate violation [are] the amount of evil to be caused, avoided, and prevented by the violation; the rational desires of the people affected by the violation; and the effect that this kind of violation, if allowed, would have.[24]

The principles of violation are similar in content to the principles by which the rules were justified in the first place, but since they have a separate place in the decision-making process, they become a mediating element in concrete moral reasoning.

Gert's ten rules are:[25]

1. Don't kill.
2. Don't cause pain.
3. Don't disable.
4. Don't deprive of freedom or opportunity.
5. Don't deprive of pleasure.
6. Don't deceive.
7. Keep your promise.

8. Don't cheat.
9. Obey the law.
10. Do your duty.

The elements of Gert's method of justification of moral rules other than negative utilitarianism are procedural -- the requirement of public agreement on the basis of rationality. This element may not itself have normative content, but it introduces mediating normative content into the reasoning process.

(5) The stages of development of Rawls's *Theory of Justice*[26] work in a similar fashion -- and thus this theory is also an example of mediation-model reasoning. The substantive rules and structures of justice which emerge at each step of the four-stage reasoning process in Rawls's *Theory* are not derived by deductive reasoning. Rather, the constraints of the "veil of ignorance" at each stage constitute a process which, combined with fundamental normative insights ("justice as fairness"), give rise to the rules appropriate to the stage in question. Thus these constraints amount to mediating elements of a mediation-model sort.

(6) Veatch's *A Theory of Medical Ethics*[27] has the same logic as Rawls's theory, upon which it builds. Indeed, the general social contract which Rawls develops forms the first of the triple contracts which Veatch develops; and it constitutes the background constraint in terms of which the second contract (i.e., that between the public as a whole as the profession as a group) is negotiated. In turn, the first and second contracts form the side constraints for negotiating the third contract between individual patients and individual professionals. At each stage, independent normative content is introduced through the negotiation and this mediates the normative force contributed by the (logically) prior contracts.

In sum, mediation-model reasoning introduces independent normative thinking to mediate the deductive process of applying theory to practice. We have offered examples from all three major ethical theories to illustrate the variations possible here. There are at least three ways in which this can be done.

First, normatively-laden definitions may be given for terms in the principles other than the deontic operators; this was illustrated by Beauchamp and Childress's second definition of "lying" in the quotation with which the chapter began. Second, indeterminacies in applying fundamental principles to the situation at hand might be eliminated by using independent normative principles to "channel the application" of fundamental principles; this is illustrated by Frankena's use of social institutions, by most forms of rule-utilitarianism, and by the Vatican *Instruction*. Third, independent normative elements (including appeals to intuition) might be referred to in order to resolve conflicts which arise between fundamental principles; the most notable exponent of this form of mediation reasoning is Sir David Ross.

E. Strengths of the Mediation Model

One of the chief strengths of the mediation model is that it can lead to agreement in practice in the face of disagreement in principle. Thinkers who approach issues from different fundamental principles can, by means of "tinkering" with the implications of their principles through mediating axioms, come to agreement on concrete issues. A celebrated (almost notorious) example of this is the position represented in Beauchamp and Childress's *Principles of Biomedical Ethics*.[28] The two authors begin from different moral theories (i.e., sets of moral principles), one from a rule-utilitarian theory and the other from an (unspecified) deontological theory; but, when they turn to analysis of concrete issues, they are in agreement on virtually every conclusion. This possibility has powerful appeal. Since fundamental issues of principle are resistant to negotiation, moral impasse is all too possible in connection with application-model reasoning (as indicated in the previous chapter). The mediation-model approach to moral reasoning offers a helpful corrective to this situation.

This approach also has the virtue of retaining much of the "flavor" (and the reality) of a deductive approach to moral reasoning. The factors that make the application-model approach appealing are also present here -- especially the rigor of argument and the linear nature of the reasoning process. The introduction of mediating principles introduces a minor aberration or anomaly in this process, but it can be viewed (a) as only a modest departure and (b) as thoroughly in the spirit of the deductive theory. The modes of inference are still thoroughly deductive -- or, at least, that is the ideal to which allegiance is still paid. The approach that would preserve the deductive character most fully would be to introduce determinate principles to play the mediating role. This is almost never done in practice; most thinkers prefer to follow Sir David Ross's dictum that "the decision rests with perception."[29] Of the examples we have reviewed, Jonsen, Siegler, and Winslade come the closest to enunciating a principle with their ranking of the four categories of considerations. However, since this ranking is only preliminary and tentative, they revert to the Rossian "situation ethics" in their analysis of concrete case examples.

The other thinkers in this camp whom we have encountered move to the Rossian model even more quickly. This approach may still retain the flavor of deductive reasoning, however, since (like Ross himself) the "perception" is interpreted as coming to understand a *principle* of priority. Thus it can still enter as a premise in a deductive syllogism (as in 3a above).

The mediation-model approach is appealing, as well, in the way it respects a certain degree of relativity; and thus offers resources for dialogue in the face of cultural pluralism and cultural variations. These can be bridged by appeal to mediating principles without the necessity for winning consensus on fundamental principles (a much more difficult task). With the proper adjustment of mediating principles, one can come to a compromise position on concrete or policy issues without having compromised one's fundamental principles.

The approach of Beauchamp and McCullough is instructive in this regard. Instead of asking physicians to abandon their historical position of beneficence (*cum* paternalism) -- as, for example, Veatch does -- they call for a balancing of this principle with a principle of autonomy (which they recognize physicians will find having a certain normative pull on their thinking already, and which they make even more palatable by interpreting it as an alternative approach to ascertaining the patient's best interests -- this from the patient's point of view). In this way, physicians need not view themselves as abandoning their historical allegiance to beneficence when they take into account the wishes of the patient. The President's Commission for the Study of Ethical Problems in Medicine and Biomedical and Behavioral Research offers an interesting similar move in its report *Making Health Care Decisions*,[30] arguing first that "promotion of a patient's well-being and respect for a patient's self-determination" are the two central values "that ought to guide decision making in the provider-patient relationship" and then attempting to reconcile these two by the claim that

> ascertaining whether a health care intervention will, if successful, promote a patient's well-being is a matter of individual judgment. Societies that respect personal freedom usually reach such decisions by leaving the judgment to the person involved.[31]

In other words, they bring in the social value of individualism and personal freedom as a mediating principle in case of conflicts between the two foundational principles.

F. Weaknesses of the Mediation Model
This approach to bridging the theory/practice gap has its difficulties, however, many of which are another way of viewing the features listed as strengths. The appearance of deductive rigor is an illusion; in actuality, this approach presents a muddle of deduction and induction. This is clearest in the forms that turn to "perception" to ascertain priorities between conflicting principles; but it also applies to forms that offer priority principles, since the origin of these is

obscure. They clearly cannot be derived from the principles on the basis of which the conflict arose (else they would not *resolve* the initial conflict). Thus they must come from some external source. At best, then, this introduces a foreign element into the theory from which the analysis began -- thus exploding its claims to the virtues of coherence and rigor; and it is likely that they stem from a form of inductive inference from the contexts, or the facts or circumstances of the situation. We will look at these forms of reasoning in later chapters. For now, however, it is sufficient to note that the inclusion of these elements into the mediating process makes the deductive approach to moral reasoning less distinct from these (usually denigrated) forms than might appear on the surface.

Unless these inductive elements are made explicit (in which case, the reasoning would have to be reclassified into one of our other categories), the approach to reasoning seems to be too formal, rigorous, and rational to apply to a process with informal, nonrigorous, and nonrational features. Pascal's dictum that "the heart has its reasons that reason cannot know" is repudiated by both application-model and mediation-model approaches. This is a basis for criticism for any who believe that Pascal offered an insight that ought to be taken into account; and the repudiation becomes ironic when it is recognized that "moves of the heart" are secretly imported into mediation model reasoning by means of priority or interpretant principles (axioms and rules).

Along with application-model reasoning, the mediation-model approach fails to offer resources for reconciling fundamental principles. Compromises, as has been indicated above, take place only at the mediation level. The original principles, and any conflicts or other discrepancies between them, remain unaltered. This is unfortunate, for it means that conflict and the consequent necessity for compromise will be a recurrent problem, whereas a reconciliation between fundamental principles (if it could be achieved) might preclude the necessity of recurrent negotiations in specific cases.

Consider Beauchamp and McCullough's approach, for example. They insist that beneficence and autonomy are likely to conflict in many situations (indeed, one is tempted to say that they "wallow" in the sense of conflict between these principles). And, since they offer no general priority principle for resolving these conflicts, their relative weight must be reexamined in each situation or type of situation. It would seem much preferable to examine the fundamental principles from which their analysis began and to attempt to reconcile these once and for all. Need beneficence lead to paternalism? Need autonomy lead to strident demands? Is not a cooperative approach possible within the framework of these two principles? These are questions which Beauchamp and McCullough do not even *ask*, much less answer. And, given their mediation-model approach, it is not hard to see why they do not address these questions. However, we will examine some thinkers who do address them; and, if they can succeed in reconciling the fundamental principles in question, the result would be a coherent approach to decision-making which would seem to be clearly preferable to the recurrent conflict and need for reconciliation through mediating principles which is characteristic of the mediation-model approach.

Although the introduction of mediating principles makes reconciliation of differences about the concrete case *possible*, it by no means makes it inevitable. There may be disagreements in interpreting middle principles, no less than fundamental principles (as we saw in the Vatican's *Instruction*); and, when "perception" is appealed to, the perceptions of the disputants may differ just as sharply as their fundamental principles. Thus, the same sort of impasse may arise at the level of middle principles, priority judgments, and the like, as we saw possible in application-model reasoning at the level of fundamental principles. If this happens, it is hard to see what resources mediation-model reasoning offers to reconcile these conflicts. Could they replicate their move with regard to fundamental principles and search for mediating principles to apply between the initial set of middle principles and the concrete case? But what if a similar sort of disagreement arises about these? One can envision a hopelessly elaborate structure of mediation soon arising like a tangle of thorns around the concrete case on which we are trying to reach agreement, making it impossible ever to come to a conclusion about what to *do*.

The most serious problem mediation-model reasoning introduces into a deductive approach to problem solving is to raise the question: Does theory really *matter*, in the last analysis? If the implications of one's fundamental principles are so readily reinterpreted (some would, of course, read this "distorted") by means of mediating principles, if deep disagreements of theory can be submerged by means of negotiation about mediating principles, then one is left to wonder what effective role moral theory or allegiance to fundamental principles really plays in moral decision-making. Moral seriousness (which has generally been defined in terms of depth of allegiance to certain fundamental principles) appears to be trivialized in the process of mediating compromise. What does it mean, for example, to say that a physician has allegiance to the historic ideal of beneficence, if this principle is frequently subordinated to autonomy in the resolution of concrete cases? Theory appears to become totally a matter of "lip service," with little relevance for action. At least the application-model theorists had the "courage of their confusions," even if we find their conclusions unpalatable and their unwillingness to compromise them illiberal.

G. Conclusion

In this chapter, we have seen that the mediation model offers the appealing possibility of resolving some of the difficulties of application-model thinking without (at least on surface analysis) giving up the deductive approach to moral reasoning. However, we saw that this surface appearance must be modified when we carefully examine the structure of this style of reasoning; and, in addition, this approach retains some of the difficulties of the application-model approach.

On all these points, we shall have to examine whether other approaches can do any better. The ideal of an approach to reasoning which offers both moral seriousness, on the one hand, and responsiveness to the concrete situation, on the other, may turn out to be an impossible ideal. But we have seen sufficient difficulties with the deductive approaches (i.e., the application model and the mediation model) to see the importance of looking at alternatives -- even if these move away from the notions of rigor, rationality, and linear thinking that many find intellectually appealing.

NOTES

1. Beauchamp and Childress, *Principles of Biomedical Ethics*, 2d ed., pp. 44-45.

2. Fried, *Right and Wrong*, p. 10.

3. Mary Anne Warren, "On the Moral and Legal Status of Abortion," *The Monist* 57, no. 1 (January 1973), 43-61.

4. Michael Tooley, "Abortion and Infanticide," *Philosophy and Public Affairs* 2, no. 1 (1972), 37-65.

5. W. D. Ross, *The Right and the Good* (Oxford: Clarendon Press, 1930), pp. 16-47.

6. Graber, Beasley, Eaddy, *Ethical Analysis of Clinical Medicine*, pp. 183-193.

7. Ibid., pp. 192-193.

8. Albert R. Jonsen, Ph.D.; Mark Siegler, M.D.; William J. Winslade, Ph.D., J.D., *Clinical Ethics: A Practical Approach to Ethical Decisions in Clinical Medicine* (New York: Macmillan, 1982), p. 6.

9. Ibid., pp. 6, 7.

10. Tom L. Beauchamp and Laurence B. McCullough, *Medical Ethics: The Moral Responsibilities of Physicians* (Englewood Cliffs, NJ: Prentice-Hall, Inc., 1984), pp. 50-51.

11. Ibid., p. 75.

12. Richard McCormick, S.J.: "Proxy Consent in the Experimentation Situation"; "Experimentation in Children: Sharing in Sociality."

13. James Rachels, "Euthanasia," in *Matters of Life and Death: New Introductory Essays in Moral Philosophy*, ed. Tom Regan (New York: Random House, 1980), pp. 28-66.

14. Ibid., p. 43.

15. Ibid., p. 53.

16. John Rawls, "Two Concepts of Rules," *Philosophical Review* 64 (1955), 3-32.

17. Congregation for the Doctrine of the Faith, *Instruction on Respect for Human Life in Its Origin and on the Dignity of Procreation* (The Vatican: Polyglot Press, 22 February 1987).

18. See also Richard McCormick, "Document Is Unpersuasive," *Health Progress* 68 (July, August 1987), 53-55.

19. David C. Thomasma, *An Apology for the Value of Human Life* (Saint Louis: The Catholic Health Association, 1983), pp. 123-124.

20. Kevin Kelly, *Life and Love* (London: Collins Liturgical Publications, 1987), p.18.

21. William K. Frankena, *Ethics*, 2nd ed. (Englewood Cliffs, NJ: Prentice-Hall, Inc., 1973), p. 54.

22. Bernard Gert, *The Moral Rules: A New Rational Foundation for Morality* (New York: Harper & Row, 1970).

23. Ibid., p. 128.

24. Ibid., pp. 125-126.

25. Ibid., p. 125.

26.   John Rawls, *A Theory of Justice* (Cambridge, MA: Harvard University Press, 1973).

27.   Veatch, *A Theory of Medical Ethics*, especially chapter 5, pp. 108-140.

28.   Beauchamp and Childress, *Principles of Biomedical Ethics*.

29. Ross, *The Right and the Good*, pp. 16-47.

30. President's Commission for the Study of Ethical Problems in Medicine and Biomedical and Behavioral Research, *Making Health Care Decisions* (Washington, DC: U.S. Government Printing Office, 1983), pp. 16-17, 41-43.

31. Ibid., pp. 41, 43.

CHAPTER FOUR
The Validation Model

The two models of reasoning we have explored so far are comfortable for and beloved by many who have turned to biomedical ethics from a background in traditional moral philosophy. However, these patterns of thought are a source of considerable frustration to clinical practitioners who explore the growing literature in biomedical ethics, as well as to the newly developing breed of clinical ethicists who seek to give full consideration to the realities in which bioethical dilemmas arise.

The difficulty can be illustrated by noting the typical reaction of dissatisfaction on the part of clinicians who read any of the popular series of "Case Studies in Bioethics"[1] that appears regularly in *The Hastings Center Report*. Each of the series consists of a case sketch describing a situation which gives rise to one or more moral dilemmas, followed by two (or sometimes three) brief analyses of the situation -- usually coming to conflicting conclusions -- by distinguished scholars in biomedical ethics. Almost invariably, these analyses consist *either* of invocation of some one fundamental ethical principle which is applied to the case in a deductive fashion to yield a conclusion about what should be done (i.e., application-model reasoning) *or else* a catalogue of two or three ethical principles which are of primary importance in dealing with the case followed by argument for giving one of these priority over the others in reaching the final conclusion about what should be done in the situation (i.e., mediation-model reasoning). These approaches are often met with disdain by clinicians because they represent modes of reasoning which in application to the clinical dimension of medical decision-making have been strongly condemned. In that context, these modes of reasoning would be labeled "cookbook medicine," a term with strongly negative overtones.

Clinical reasoning (or at least the understanding of it that is taught in contemporary medical schools and embraced by contemporary physicians) is much more pragmatic than this. Any and all general principles are held tentatively as hypotheses, and they are regularly abandoned in the maelstrom of dealing with the concrete clinical case. They are replaced by strategies suggested by the exigencies of the individual clinical situation. The received doctrine in medical practice nowadays is that each case is unique and importantly idiosyncratic, and thus that general principles cannot guide clinical practice in any but the most rudimentary way. What is emphasized is analogical rather than deductive reasoning. Hypotheses rather than principles are the rule.

Given the pluralistic cast of modern society, it is no surprise that a third model of relating theory and practice in medical ethics has gained impetus over the past ten years. This model views the goal of reasoning in biomedical ethics to be *policies* -- something a bit more general than a decision for the particular case (since they are meant to deal "with a set of situations which create a similar type of problem"[2]) but not so general or settled as a rule or principle. General moral principles (including those on the highest level, such as the principle of utility or a Kantian principle of respect for persons) are viewed rather as act-utilitarians view moral rules (but not the principle of utility itself) -- that is, as rough-and-ready generalizations of past exercises in policy formulation. Terrence Ackerman amplifies this point when he says of moral policies, "They summarize the wisdom of past efforts to deal with concrete moral problems."[3] The criterion of a justified policy, in Ackerman's view, is one that "effectively achieves the body of aims which the persons involved would choose with adequate knowledge of the situation or set of situations in question,"[4] and in this way ethical theory is validated by practice through the establishment of either moral policy or practical decisions guided by the procedural goal of respecting as many moral elements in a case as possible.

A. Examples of Validation Model Reasoning

(1) It stands to reason that, as exasperated health professionals, policy planners, lawyers, and politicians attempt to resolve the difficult medico-moral quandaries of our time, they would turn to any and all proposals for constructing a reasonable and pragmatic synthesis of values. Consider, for example, the Catholic hospital in an inner-city neighborhood. Its Ob-Gyn department, composed mostly of non-Catholic physicians, serves an overwhelmingly non-Catholic population. The Catholic hospital staff wishes it to stand as a commitment of service to the poor. This value is shared by diocesan officials as well. Its board, whose membership is mostly non-Catholic, believes in this commitment but more as a vital service to the community than as a specifically *Catholic* institutional task. Society itself has relevant concerns as well, including holding down health care costs, protecting against child abuse, lowering the teenage pregnancy rate, and keeping population growth under control. Social values like these, incorporated into and supplemented by the personal values of a welfare mother, might (and sometimes does) lead her to request

sterilization. In one sense, not to provide a response to this request violates many values. To provide this service, on the other hand, would run counter to current Catholic teaching and practice on the value of human life.

To single out one or a few elements of this situation and relate them to determinate principles in a linear, deductive fashion would be a gross oversimplification and distortion of the complexities of this concrete moral situation. What is needed is an approach that incorporates an appreciation for *all* the values involved and that attempts to reconcile conflicts between them as much as possible. In short, what is needed is a way to make the best of an admittedly less-than-ideal situation. "Compromise" is not a category of deductive reasoning, nor is "negotiation," nor "creative synthesis." From the point of view of application-model reasoning, these approaches to developing a policy amount to *abandoning* the principles in question. The attempt to preserve and respect the "spirit" of the principle, which is central to the process of policy validation is opaque from the application-model perspective.

This case is but one of thousands which exemplify the typical form medical ethics problems take in our time. It poses a challenge of priorities between a mixture of diverse goods (and evils) rather than a choice between clear-cut good on one hand and evil on the other. Among the hidden assumptions of validation-model reasoning are (a) the notion that earlier ethical theories (such as those proposed by Aristotle, Aquinas, the Scottish commonsense philosophers, Locke, Kant, and to some extent Mill) were all formulated in an age in which ethics dealt with choices between good and evil, and (b) consequently that these theories can no longer provide answers in an age like ours, which is preoccupied with choosing among competing goods -- while, ironically, eschewing the kind of metaphysical thinking necessary to validate such choices.

Of course, if the hidden assumptions were to be fully articulated and defended, these assumptions would appear somewhat naive. Conflicts among goods, not just between good and evil, are part and parcel of these earlier ethical theories, from Socrates' final struggle between the truth of his own conscience and the common good of justice, through Mill's utilitarianism itself. Nonetheless, validation-model proponents may have a basis for charging that the resources of those earlier theories are less than fully adequate to resolve the complex conflicts among competing social, individual, professional, and personal goods presented by modern culture.[5]

Richard McCormick characterizes the contemporary Catholic moral tradition in very similar terms, arguing that the shift in approach was tied in with Vatican II and is illustrated most clearly by the relation of laypersons to social teachings.

John [XXIII] moved from the deductive to the inductive method, his point of departure being the "historical moment" to be viewed in light of the Gospel. This led to a complete reevaluation of the place of laypersons vis-à-vis social teachings, a reevaluation completed by Vatican II. Laypersons do not simply apply the Church's social teaching; they must share in its very construction.[6]

Speaking more directly of method, McCormick says:

Catholic tradition is always innovative and, in a sense, always in flux. In its task of "formation of consciousness," it takes seriously the findings of human experience and human sciences. Its method is necessarily inductive. That means that it will at times necessarily say things that were not said before, and even modify things that were said before. It will not hesitate to be exploratory and tentative.[7]

McCormick's claim that current realities must be viewed "in light of the Gospel" shows that fundamental norms play a significant role in his understanding of moral reasoning. Thus, in spite of his terminology, his is not a purely inductive model as we would characterize it. However, he classifies earlier ways at arriving at the Church's social teaching as examples of application-model reasoning and criticizes them on much the same basis as our criticisms of the application model.

Joseph Fletcher has also recently proclaimed allegiance to an inductive model and we would also classify his model as validation-model reasoning. He dismisses the application-model approach on epistemological grounds: "as a matter of *cognition*, we cannot establish a theory first and then proceed to cases."[8] He describes the approach he favors in these terms:

To be sound, ethical theory, like all other kinds of theory, must be born out of experiences with actual problems. It is experimental, empirical, and data based; a posteriori, not a priori. Moral rules and principles ought to be empirical generalizations, changeable when experience changes, not rigid laws but more like the prima facie guidelines that W. D. Ross expounded -- at first sight obliging but sometimes not always so on a second look.[9]

The last sentence makes it clear that he is not proposing a purely inductive model. Instead of dispensing with general norms, as a pure inductive model requires, Fletcher proposes subjecting pre-existing moral rules to validation through concrete, situational moral experience.

(2) A short story by Richard Selzer provides a dramatic glimpse of these value-conflict levels. The doctor enters the room of a dying

patient.   A halting dialogue eventually reveals the patient's request
that the doctor end his pain and suffering, and the doctor's refusal
for reasons of conscience.   But is the refusal really based on
conscience?   As he returns to the hallway, he realizes in the depth
of his being, with clinical detail, that he has betrayed the patient
because, as a physician and as a person, he is a coward. He learns
that the limits of his usual commitment to act in the best interests
of patients have been set into stark relief by this one instance.[10]

If patients develop a bond with doctors, and as that bond
encourages them to struggle with their own moral values as essential
elements of autonomy, then the days will come increasingly when
patients will ask for active euthanasia.[11]   At that moment, the
heartrending lineup of goods sears the very soul of a health
professional. On the one hand there are values such as commitment
to preserve life, to do no harm, legal prohibitions, fears about
destroying one's family, jail, etc. On the other hand are marshaled
the values of encouraging patient autonomy, loyalty, desire not to
abandon the patient when one can offer nothing medically but
palliation, a commitment to relief of suffering, and (if the physician
has come to see what Selzer's has) facing up to one's own conscience
and acting on it.

Within this snapshot from a doctor's life, then, are value clashes
on all levels, from personal through professional and institutional, to
social, legal, and cultural.   These occur (a) internally, within each
participant (one can very well imagine the value struggle a patient
must transverse to make such a request as a serious gesture of finality
and recognition of the futility of one's life), (b) between participants,
and (c) between all these parties and the standard interests of the
state in protecting the lives of its citizens.   There are too many
important values in this real-life drama for a soap-opera resolution.
As the doctor staggers from the room, his life has been altered. This
profound new self-recognition must eventually lead to new conduct, to
new social institutions, to new policies.

The thought process which has these results is one example of
validation-model thinking. It is unlikely that this physician will focus
on some one or a few central principles from which to perform
deductions.   Furthermore, it is even more unlikely that he or she
would find this procedure helpful. Instead, the physician will attempt
first to identify and then to sort through the myriad values which
have arisen in this incident.

(3) Within the past twenty years literally hundreds of panels have
been created to press forward the task of resolving ethical issues
through the creation of policy. The most enduring of these, and the
ones most likely to have a long-term impact are the Institutional
Review Boards[12] which determine whether a given research project

adequately protects policy guidelines (or policy conclusions), and newly forming hospital ethics committees[13] which attempt to formulate and implement moral policy with respect to clinical cases arising in hospitals (such as treatment decisions for defective newborns[14] or for comatose but not brain-dead patients[15]). We can only mention here some of the many other important panels which have formulated policy recommendations on such problems as determining the moment of death,[16] establishing hospital ethics committees,[17] *in utero* fetal surgery,[18] resource allocation and implanting artificial hearts,[19] and surrogate motherhood and *in vitro* fertilization.[20]

If formulating moral policy were merely a matter of deducing the implications for the situation at hand from abstract principles, all these groups could be replaced by a few skilled logicians working individually. The fact that various agencies and groups are drawn to form panels, then, is a tacit endorsement of the much less determinate and more person-dependent and interdisciplinary validation-model patterns of reasoning. (The point of assembling a *group* of persons, of course, is to cancel out biases which might be introduced due to this person-dependent aspect through negotiation among diverse individuals.)

(4) Indeed, the President's Commission for the Study of Ethical Problems in Medicine and Biomedical and Behavioral Research recommends development of a policy precisely *in lieu of* a clear conclusion in the primary situation. This is exemplified by the following excerpt from the commission's report, "Deciding to Forego Life-Sustaining Treatment":

> Hospitals should have an explicit policy on the practice of writing and implementing DNR orders. In the absence of an established mechanism, decisionmaking might fail to meet the requirements of informed consent or the responsibility for making and carrying out the decision might be assigned to an inappropriate person. Physicians should be allowed to decide to stop a resuscitation effort in progress, although the authority of inexperienced or untrained individuals to make such a decision should be limited. Moreover, without a deliberate process for reaching decisions about resuscitation, legitimate options may never receive the full consideration of patients, physicians, and other involved parties. Consultations with the nursing staff might well be required.[21]

Here consensus and the importance of clearly stated procedures (admittedly not directly relevant to the substantive issue at hand) are offered as *substitutes* for substantive, normative guidelines, since it seems to be taken for granted that agreement is not possible on which conclusions could be deduced from established principles. This seems to be a perfect illustration of Alasdair MacIntyre's dictum that preoccupation with procedure accompanies a breakdown of agreement on substantive values and ethical principles.[22]

(5) The importance of policy as a means of determining ethical principles and solving what become ethico-political issues is underscored by Daniel Callahan in his Shattuck Lecture of 1980.[23] Callahan argues that, compared to the difficult task of establishing ethical policies in medicine, case analysis and resolution is relatively simple. The reason, he claims, is that case resolution is often limited to the relatively few parties directly involved, while establishing ethical policy becomes a political process, combining the components of analysis with a synthetic task which is constantly at risk of being skewed by values other than ethical ones.

(6) Arthur Dyck argued in the early days of medical ethics that in addition to principles and axioms in medical ethics, one needs moral policy as well.[24] The reason is that such policy can help tailor ethics towardsmore practical concerns. He argues that medical ethics must include a descriptive, a normative, and a policy component. The idea of moral policy is to establish guidelines for action in which theories are incorporated into an action plan. Dyck does not claim that theories arise from practice (as origination-model proponents claim); rather he suggests that conflicting theories are somehow reconciled in the policy. The fact that he holds a position at Harvard University Medical School in which he is responsible for articulating ideas for population policy makes his appeal for more attention to this element of ethics all the more important. In his *On Human Care*, published slightly later than the essay cited previously, he follows Ralph Potter in defining moral policy as:

> Recommendations for what should be done here and now . . . specifying a responsible agent, a goal, and an appropriate means for its realization.[25]

But how would such policy development actually differ from an application-model process like that described in chapter 2, whereby one moves from principles (such as respect for persons) to policy conclusions (such as forbidding research on children) through intermediate steps? The difference lies in the process of reasoning, which includes many more steps (each less precise than in straightforward deductive reasoning) and many more principles at once. One does not so much "deduce" policies from principles as try to fit the principles together into an acceptable framework. Prior reasoning, as we shall show, may proceed deductively, however. This gives rise to the name we give one branch of the deductive process: *validation*, because the theory developed is validated by (or, in some positions, the theory even derives its truth from) its pragmatic consequences. The policy's effects in practice validate the theory or (more often) theories joined in the policy.

There are at least two forms of this logical process. In the first, one or more prior theories are appealed to in the process of identifying and sorting through the myriad moral elements in the situation of choice. In some cases, these prior theories may be approved unchanged as a result of the reconciliation process -- in which case, we can say that the theories have been *validated* by concrete moral experience. In other cases, the prior theories will be further defined and/or altered in this process -- in which case, we can say that the theory is determined (at least in part) by the process of concrete moral decision-making.

In the other form of this process, prior theoretical principles play a relatively minor role. Policies are determined more by the exigencies, moral insights, and moral negotiations in the concrete situation of choice than by any abstract prior theoretical commitments. (This forms the matter of the next chapter.)

(7) In the first form, the differences between deductive and mediated models and validation models is one of degree, not kind. The reasoning in validation is simply more complex, and one does not stop with middle-level axioms, but moves on to policy formulation. A good example of this is provided by an earlier work of Robert Veatch, *Death, Dying, and the Biological Revolution.*[26] In this work Veatch was concerned with shoring up the rights of persons to "manage" their own death, to decide whether or not they wished to have certain therapies and treatments, and to die with dignity. He therefore argued to this middle level axiom: patients have a right to refuse treatment. But he did so by examining a host of issues, rather than by a linear deductive process from some one or a few foundational principles. The bare bones logic might look like 4a.

In order to focus on key elements, we have left out a number of steps in the argument -- such as the legal interpretation needed to validate the axiom that patients have a right to refuse treatment as an expression of autonomy and the right to privacy or the descriptive research about present institutional realities required to validate the call for a new policy by physicians. Appeal must be made, not to logical entailments of the principle of death with dignity itself, but to practices in the community -- court cases, paternalistic decisions made for dying patients, and the like. It is these social and clinical realities which validate the move from principle to policy conclusion, interpreting both the content of autonomy for today's health-care practice and the classes of persons to whom the principle applies.

(8) An especially clear example of the nonlinear nature of this process is seen in the gradual formulation by the United States Supreme Court of the constitutional right to privacy. First discovered

---

4a

Moral theory:	Respect for Persons
Legal theory:	Legal Doctrine of the Right to Privacy
Moral principle:	Persons have a fundamental right to autonomy or self-determination.
Descriptive factors:	Significant court cases can be interpreted as taking this right to mean that persons have a right to refuse treatment.
Axiomatic conclusion:	Patients have an autonomous right to refuse treatment, especially when they are dying.
Normative premise:	This right takes precedence over the physician's duties to preserve life.
Practical conclusion:	Physicians should have little or no say about a patient's decision to die.
Descriptive factors:	Current practices in clinical institutions leave the patient little say in decisions about their death.
Indicated course of action:	Hence, physicians ought to make special efforts to respect a dying patient's request. (Death with dignity)

---

in 1964 lurking in the "penumbra" of the U. S. Constitution, it has been applied by state supreme courts to a progressively wider sphere of cases in ensuing years.[27] Richard Nixon was correct when he said that this sort of reasoning hardly amounts to "strict construction" (i.e., linear deduction). His mistake was in thinking that such an alternative approach to legal interpretation was even *possible*, much less *desirable*.

(9) A further example demonstrates the use of deductive reasoning in reaching a decision about the complexity of policy. This example shows how practical concerns and descriptive research data enter further into the deductive process, inescapably leading to an awareness that one cannot proceed purely deductively (deriving a conclusion from one principle) as in the models outlined in previous chapters. In order to underline this point, the example first shows a deductive process at work, then brings in the validation model.

Consider the ethical reasoning about artificial insemination by a donor (AID) for single women. Many women today, either by choice, happenstance, or sexual preference, do not get married. Yet some of these women would like to have children. Is it proper for specialists in Ob-Gyn to help them towards that goal by inseminating them with donor sperm? Arguments *against* such a procedure might take the (application-model) form of 4b.[28]

4b

Normative premise: In considering AID, the dominant and inescapable interest must be that of the child.

Descriptive premise: But a father-absent household jeopardizes the best interests of the child.

Practical conclusion: Hence a father-absent household disrupts the dominant and inescapable interests to be considered with regard to AID.

A second (also deductive) form of the argument against AID for single women focuses on the duty of a physician.*

4c

Normative premise: The first duty of a physician in considering AID is the best interests of the child. The desire of a patient to have a child must remain merely a subordinate interest.

Descriptive premise: But a father-absent household (as would be the case in lives of lesbians, divorcees who do not remarry, and those who have participated in Doonesbury's "singleness ceremony"*) jeopardizes the best interests of the child.

Practical conclusion: Therefore the first duty of a physician considering AID is violated by a father-absent household.

Of course, in both forms of this deductive argument, the minor (descriptive) premise is especially vulnerable. To defend it one argues that children in father-absent homes are bound to be adversely affected by sex-role modeling, by social ostracism if the parent is publicly labeled as a lesbian or cohabitates with a lesbian partner, by the lack of stability in nonstandard relationships, and by poor cognitive and social development if the mother works (since the bond between mother and child, especially in the early formative years, would be less qualitatively satisfactory than in a dual-parent home).

An awareness of the need for better data regarding the minor premise can lead to a recognition that other principles ought also to be used in the major, thus leading to the use of the "validation" model.

---

* The ritual of a singleness ceremony was celebrated during July and August 1985 in the syndicated "Doonesbury" comic strip in newspapers throughout the United States.

Strong and Schinfeld[29] argue against ruling out AID for single women in all instances, using arguments we would classify in the validation model. Note that their argument begins from the same major premise as the argument *against* AID for single women. In schematic form, their reasoning looks like 4d.

4d

Normative premise: The first duty of a physician in considering AID for a single woman is the best interests of the child.

Descriptive factor: But the data about how father-absent homes affect the best interests of the child are ambiguous.

Conclusion: The first duty of a physician in considering AID is to respect the ambiguity of the data.

Descriptive premise: But respecting the ambiguity of the data means to decide on a case-by-case basis under the guidance of policy.

Practical Conclusion: The first duty of a physician in considering AID, then, is to decide on a case-by-case basis under the direction of policy.

Note, now, how the conclusion returns to the original major premise and alters it. *Validation* is a process of reasoning, that leads deductively from a major premise through descriptively-based minors (rather than axiomatically-derived normative statements) to a conclusion that actually alters the major. In our example, the final conclusion states that physicians have no *single* duty to protect the potential child, but rather a duty to consider a number of factors. The policy to be developed would offer a checklist of considerations to be taken into account. Strong and Schinfeld list the following:

» the health of the recipient;
» her financial situation;
» the presence of an extended family or other probabilities that child-adult counseling will take place;
» the recipient's support system;
» how maturely the recipient thought through the forthcoming difficulties; and
» the presence of the donor's informed consent about single parenting.

Defense of the minor takes the form of balancing the value of existing over not existing at all, or the value of existing in a parent-absent environment over not existing, both of which are weighted in favor of existing. The new major premise (the conclusion about case-by-case policy) is supported by pointing out that physicians do not practice in an ideal chamber, but in the real world.   In addition, the interests of the mother cannot be totally dismissed from consideration.

In this approach, the physician is not obligated to offer AID in every case, since AID is neither a medical treatment nor a health-related need of the woman.   There is no single moral principle from which indicated courses of action are to be deduced.   Finally, reasonable guidelines or policies like those proposed function as a protection for physicians in "wrongful life" suits, since it can be demonstrated that the physician rested judgment on a set of objective standards rather than subjective preferences open to the charge of being prejudicial.

In the Veatch example (4a above), the theory of respect for persons and the moral principle of autonomy are accepted without adjustment.   The validation consists of interpreting the principle and applying it to the situation at hand.   But in 4d, Strong and Schinfeld have actually altered the normative premise by adjusting it, validating their new principle in light of social realities.

(10) Consider another example of moral theory being validated by practice.   It stems from the compromise "Baby Doe" amendment to child abuse legislation in 1983.   The policy mandated state child protective services agencies to investigate instances of "medical neglect" including "withholding medically indicated treatment from disabled infants with life-threatening conditions."   The policy defines withholding "medically indicated treatment" as:

> The failure to respond to the infant's life-threatening conditions by providing treatment (including appropriate nutrition, hydration, and medication) which, in the treating physician's or physicians' reasonable medical judgment, will most likely be effective in ameliorating or correcting all such conditions; the term does not include failure to provide treatment (other than appropriate nutrition, hydration, or medication) when, in the treating physician's or physicians' reasonable medical judgment, (a) the infant is chronically and irreversibly comatose; (b) the provision of such treatment would (i) merely prolong dying, (ii) not be effective in ameliorating or correcting all the infant's life-threatening conditions, or (iii) otherwise be futile in terms of the survival of the infant; or (c) the provision of such treatment would be virtually futile in terms of the survival of the infant and the treatment itself would be inhumane.[30]

This policy was already the result of intense national debate about the constitutional rights of defective newborns to life and the discretionary judgments of families and physicians.   This was at least the third set of "Baby Doe Rules" to be issued by the federal government (Reagan administration), the first two having been struck down by courts. In its unmodified form, it seems to imply that food, water, and medications should never be withheld even from dying infants. As many ethicists and medical bodies such as the American Academy of Pediatrics were quick to point out, the policy had the result of unduly prolonging the dying of some defective newborns. It was therefore further modified in 1984, as a result of a wide-ranging political compromise.[31]

The policy was not the result of deductive reasoning from a single principle or set of principles, though it was no less clearly an "ethical"* policy than one that might have been so derived. Instead notice was given that the judgment of inhumane treatment in the policy would depend on experimentation and experience with major technological interventions and selecting from among them only those that would achieve the goal(s) sought.

Further, the conflicting moral theories and principles which figured into this negotiation were numerous. The policy had to respect all these principles insofar as possible:

» the constitutional right to life;
» the rights of children;
» nonmaleficence;
» parental rights to decide treatment questions for their children;
» physician duties to preserve life and determine appropriate treatments (the axiom of medical indications);
» the duty of the state to protect the lives of its citizens;
» the hard-won rights to equal treatment for the retarded;
» the use of expensive and contested resources;
» the obligation not to prolong dying; and
» the need to allow for professional discretionary judgment regarding patients whose treatment is most likely futile.

Any one of these principles could function by itself in a deductive scheme; but these schemes would lead to widely divergent practical conclusions.

Hence the policy itself represents an attempt to affirm a number of principles simultaneously. Testing took place in the political forum. One significant impetus towards modification occurred when a consequence was noted about food, water, and medication which

---

* which is not to say it was ethically *correct* -- the contrast is with "nonethical," rather than "unethical."

seemed to violate current standards in treating adults. As a consequence of the debate, certain major principles were modified, as in example 4d. Discretionary space for physicians was kept intact but circumscribed to the domain of useless treatment. Society's interest in protecting the lives of its citizens was not extended to the realm of futile treatments which would offer only short-term extension of life. Parental judgment was also limited.

In the validation model, the goal of reasoning is the creation of policy. Principles are viewed as generalizations incorporating past experience in policy formation and thus potentially modifiable through current and future experience. Hence they have no independent normative bite apart from policies in which they are balanced and checked against one another.

(11) One of the ways policy formulation can go wrong is by focusing exclusively on a single principle and failing to note the moral complexities in the situation of choice. This, in our judgment, is the root error in the 1987 action of the Illinois legislature in passing a conscience law which permits physicians to fail to inform patients at risk for having a child with birth defects of the availability of prenatal diagnosis. Honoring conscience is, indeed, an important value -- but there are also other important values in this situation, including informed consent and the underlying principle of autonomy/respect for persons, parental privacy or discretion, and standards of good medical care, as well as the right to life of the fetus. As critics of the proposed law point out in a newspaper editorial:

> At its irreducible core, medical ethics teaches physicians to do no harm. House Bill 1415 . . . authorizes them to do harm to their patients -- by failing to warn them of possible genetic problems and to explain the diagnostic and treatment options available.[32]

The argument of those who want the new legislation is interesting as well. It runs as follows. Additional "conscience" legislation is important because the standard legislation is inadequate to protect properly those physicians who refuse to treat someone from a malpractice suit. If a physician refuses to perform an amniocentesis, for example, because she suspects her patient would abort the fetus if it were discovered to be either defective, or even the "wrong" sex, proponents of the new legislation argue that the physician would remain unprotected from the patient's legal ire.

The argument runs as shown in 4e.

Thus the argument[33] hinges on the question of whether or not the life of a handicapped or defective fetus can be considered to be wrongful. The problem with the legislation as proposed is that some defects are worse than others, and that therefore, some physician

4e

Major premise:	Handicapped fetuses, like handicapped persons, must be protected from eugenic killing.
Minor Premise:	Eugenic abortion is a form of eugenic killing.
Conclusion:	Handicapped fetuses require protection from eugenic abortion.

Major premise:	Handicapped fetuses require protection from eugenic abortion.
Minor premise:	Such protection can be provided by physicians who refuse to act on the request of the mother for abortion on the basis of their conscience.
Conclusion:	Therefore conscientious withdrawal can protect the lives of handicapped fetuses.
Argument for the minor:	Current conscience laws are insufficient to protect the physician who refuses to participate in a decision to abort a defective fetus. They are insufficient because, in the words of one spokesperson, "proponents of eugenic abortion...would like to single out such abortions and force medical personnel to assist such abortions under penalty of a 'wrongful birth' lawsuit, even if they conscientiously object to abortions."

refusals are more directly an abandonment of duties than others. The best possible policy is one that best respects important values in the practice of medicine. In this case it strikes us as most important to protect the conscience of individuals as well as the rights and responsibilities of those who are pregnant, as well as those who care for them. It seems best to rely on previous conscience legislation (since one cannot protect completely from lawsuits) to cover the conscientious withdrawal from care on the part of physicians without underlining their potential abandonment of patients. In other words, the additional legislation, as social policy, might provide too much protection at the expense of individuals who need care.

(12) It is a mark of the maturity of medical ethics to recognize that no one principle can predominate in practice. Consider a recent alteration of viewpoint by James Childress in this regard. We have already mentioned his deontological stand and his meta-ethical choice of rights over goods, of autonomy over beneficence.[34] Nonetheless, in discussing care, respect, and fairness for the elderly, he notes:

> It is not time to repudiate autonomy unless it is wrongly conceived as the single, exclusive, or overriding principle of biomedical ethics. What is needed is a richer portrayal of several principles and their

relationships, along with the images and metaphors that shape our policies.[35]

If Childress had merely spoken of developing priority judgments to reconcile conflicts between autonomy and other principles, we would classify his reasoning as an example of the mediation model.[*] However, his recognition of the role of "images and metaphors [which] shape our policies" brings him squarely into validation-model forms of reasoning. The argument Childress constructs could be represented as shown in 4f and 4g.[**][36]

4f

Normative premise:	The right to health care stems from two principles, beneficence (compassion) and justice (fairness).
Descriptive premise:	Illness and disease in old age stem from the natural lottery that is seen either as unfortunate (compassion) or as unfair (fairness).
Conclusion:	Hence old age and its illnesses seem to intercept naturally the right to health care.

4g

Normative premise:	Old age and its illnesses can naturally intercept the right to health care.
Descriptive premise:	The right to health care can be abridged on the basis of two axioms (what we call rules) to be specified below.
Policy conclusion:	Elders can have limits set on their care based on these two axioms (rules).

---

[*] Note that his original position -- with its linear arguments from the single principle of autonomy to conclusions for specific cases -- is an instance of application-model reasoning.

[**] Norman Daniels (see n. 36) argues that age-discrimination is not like other forms of discrimination because it lies not *between* lives but within a life. All persons will age.

In Childress's suggested policy the rules of limitation are that (a) one has no obligation to offer care that has no reasonable benefit, and -- more controversially -- (b) there is no obligation to provide care if costs outweigh benefits. Hence, expensive life-sustaining technologies can be denied because they violate one of the two rules and thus are not synonymous with offering communal care. This point has also been raised by the Office of Technology Assessment of the United States Congress in its report on "Life-Sustaining Technologies and the Elderly."[37] Of interest to the argument is the way in which deductive reasoning is still employed even though two principles and two rules are used to develop a policy. Unlike application-model or mediation-model reasoning, however, no one principle predominates, as per Childress's own reflections on this point.

Aging patients are often discriminated against precisely because of their age. By now, the statement imputed to former Governor Lamm of Colorado is well-known: "Old people have a duty to die and get out of the way." This is a form of ageism that is abhorrent to medical practice. If public policy is to be dominated by age as a criterion in health care, it must be known ahead of time to all, and all persons, upon reaching a certain age and denied access to some form of health care, must be treated alike.[38]

To base public policy on the single principle of age destroys human freedom. It is sacrificed to expediency and social efficiency. Thus, Mark Siegler argues against age as an independent criterion in health care because it violates the nature of the doctor-patient relationship (4h).

4h	
Major premise:	An essential feature of the doctor-patient relationship is discrimination (judging the proportion between therapy and prognosis).
Minor premise:	In an age of expediency rather than morality, discrimination is destroyed by considering external factors such as the age of the patient.
Conclusion:	Current public policy of expediency destroys the doctor-patient relationship.

To support his minor premise, Siegler argues that from Hippocrates until 1965, during the Age of Paternalism, there was a correct perception of medically indicated treatment. The doctors made the decisions. From 1965 until October 1, 1983, Siegler claims, the Age of Paternalism was succeeded by the Age of Autonomy: an appreciation of the patient's values and preferences. October 1, 1983 ushered in a new era, the Age of Bureaucratic Parsimony, when Diagnosis Related Groups (DRGs) were inaugurated. These introduced factors such as the quality of life of the patient, curtailing hospital costs, and the like, that have destroyed the discriminatory powers of medicine acting for the good of the patient.

In place of this public policy, Siegler argues that there should be one that:

1. maintains and promotes discriminatory judgment in the doctor-patient relation;
2. demands quality of care in traditional medical terms; and
3. if we are to ration, begins with the strongest and most articulate first.[39]

The problem with this approach to public policy is that all previous forms of health care in the United States discriminated against those who could not pay (often the poor and the aged).[40] Even though Siegler argues that everyone has a right to health care (a claim with which we are in sympathy), it is hard to conceive how this program could be carried out in light of escalating costs.

(13) A good example of the dangers of resolving ethical dilemmas by appeal to policy can be found in problems associated with the AIDS crisis. As is now the case, there are efforts by society to control the disease, and therefore to limit the autonomy of individuals in favor of the general well-being of all. In addition, there are well-defined issues of protecting confidentiality, providing insurance and other coverage for those afflicted with the disease, and protecting health-care workers from potentially death-dealing contact with the blood and other bodily fluids of carriers of the disease. The problem of how to handle health care workers who have the disease, or are HIV positive, has also surfaced.

The Centers for Disease Control in Atlanta issued guidelines in this regard, the gist of which is to stress that AIDS, unlike other serious infectious diseases, cannot be passed on except through intimate sexual contact, exchange of fluids, or sharing of needles. Although no one is willing to claim that there is *no chance at all* of someone contracting the disease from casual contact, the chances are in fact so slim as to be on an order of magnitude of thousandths compared to the chance of a patient contracting some other infectious disease from a health professional, a disease such as hepatitis.

As a consequence, the CDC guidelines appear to protect individual health care workers who contract the disease from any undue discrimination. There is no basis in the guidelines, for example, for removing a physician so infected from the care of patients just on the basis of that physician having the disease.[41] Instead, the CDC recommends dealing with each case on an individual basis through standard hospital mechanisms available for judging physician impairments. Most specialists in infectious diseases agree with these guidelines, as do other physicians.

Yet there are other interests that ought to be protected in general social policies. Two additional interests came to light in a case that appeared at Cook County hospital in Chicago. A young physician contracted AIDS. Once this became apparent, he was initially removed from patient-care responsibilities and given an administrative position. When he protested, this decision was revoked, and he was given limited patient-care and teaching responsibilities. He tried to treat patients under these restrictions, but after several days, voluntarily removed himself from their care on the grounds that he could not practice his discipline at the level of the standards of care required. Simultaneous with the original removal, he began a process of appeal with the help of the American Civil Liberties Union. In the view of the latter organization, his removal from patient care responsibilities violated antidiscrimination laws against the handicapped and caused him to sever important bonds between doctor and patient.

By giving him a different position within the hospital, the administration argued that there was no loss of salary or benefits, particularly health insurance. The normal appeals process within the institution brought out the following set of complex issues not at that time covered in the Centers for Disease Control's policy, nor for that matter, covered by the particular employee policies of most health care institutions.[42]

- AIDS as a handicap: Rulings of courts regarding students who were removed from school had established the notion that AIDS was a handicap. But could a physician make this claim about the disease and argue that his removal from patient care was a form of discrimination?
- Do physicians have a right to practice that is so intrinsic to their profession that only documented and real harms to patients are sufficient grounds to revoke their right?
- Can a hospital board, acting to protect patients from even the most remote harm, revoke the patient-care privileges of a physician?

- If so, then should all current and future employees of the hospital be screened for the HIV virus? If many test positive, and all must have jobs within the institution, will there be enough administrative posts to go around?
- Would a policy of revoking patient-care privileges on the remotest chance of infection be wise, considering the much more dramatic chance of contracting other life-threatening illnesses from hospitals and hospital staff personnel?
- Is the fear of catching AIDS from one's doctor or nurse irrational? Is it not rational to choose the 1 percent chance of contracting a disease that is potentially curable (Hepatitis-B for example) over the 0.001 percent chance of contracting a disease that is always fatal? Is it not, in fact, reasonable for persons to choose the safest environment? Do patients have a right to such an environment when they enter hospitals?
- Do patients have a right to know that their health professional has HIV-positive disease? After all, physicians and nurses demand to know if their patient has the disease.
- Should health professionals voluntarily disclose the fact that they have AIDS to patients in an effort to educate them that the disease cannot be passed on through casual contact?
- What are the duties of institutions towardsworkers who do disclose this information, voluntarily or by law? Clearly they should not fire them, or otherwise destroy their health benefits and standing in the community. But what about counseling, protection of their confidentiality, or compassion?
- If health professionals are removed from full or partial patient-care responsibilities, does this convey a message to those health professionals who refuse to treat AIDS patients? The message might be that, although all scientific evidence points to the fact that AIDS cannot be contracted through casual contact, properly protected health professionals may still pass AIDS on to patients. Consequently, those who refuse to treat AIDS patients may be legitimately concerned that AIDS might be passed on to them inadvertently as well.

These and other questions that arise in such cases demonstrate that a policy of either total removal from patient care and/or invasive procedures on the one hand, or a commitment to complete patient-care responsibilities on the other, are doomed to fail. Whatever policy is developed ought to safeguard the common good (minimizing any possible risk to patients) while underscoring a compassionate commitment to the individual health professional. This is a very difficult challenge.

(14) Two other even more obvious examples of policies which have been forged from often-intense professional and public debate are the report of the AMA Judicial Council on patient preferences and

terminal illness, and court responses to withdrawing fluids and nutrition. Let us examine each of these in turn.

The AMA Judicial Council policy represents an official departure from the time-tested responses embodied in physician paternalism. If any argument were ever advanced for such paternalism, it might look like the application-model reasoning in 4i.

4i

Major principle: Beneficence (acting in the best interests of the patient) is the
                        primary duty of the physician.

Descriptive premise: But a doctor knows what is best for dying patients.

Policy conclusion: Beneficence requires that doctors make decisions in the best
                        interests of dying patients.

Defense of the minor, descriptive premise often involves anecdotal stories of patients who either asked physicians to make decisions for them or made inappropriate requests out of ignorance, fear, or some other impediment to voluntary, free decision-making. In fact, arguments about the matter in the minor premise require alteration of Robert Veatch's strong position on autonomy and self-determination (i.e., argument 4a). Persons are not *always* the best judge of their own good.

The AMA policy differs from argument 4a by taking this fact into account, and by including (salvaging actually) some role for the physician vis-à-vis the decisions of a dying patient -- while nevertheless affirming the undeniable right of patients to make their own decisions:

> A competent, adult patient may, in advance, formulate and provide a valid consent to the withholding or withdrawal of life-support systems in the event that injury or illness renders that individual incompetent to make such a decision. The preference of the individual should prevail when determining whether extraordinary life-prolonging measures should be undertaken in the event of terminal illness. Unless it is clearly established that the patient is irreversibly, terminally ill, a physician should not be deterred from appropriately aggressive treatment of a patient.[43]

Note how different this policy is from one developed from argument 4a (Veatch's argument) or argument 4i (the paternalism argument). Policies, in order to be acceptable to both patients and physicians, must protect what President Franklin Roosevelt once called "a concert of interests." We saw, in the example of the "Baby Doe" regulations, that policies are inevitably forged from compromises. Of course, individual bureaucracies and institutions may still churn out policies that protect only their own interests. But in the national bio-ethics arena, such self-serving attempts are simply not viable. Once a moral policy must be designed to protect more than one value, then the validation process begins. In the case of the AMA policy, the physician's duties (a) to preserve life, (b) to treat a disease aggressively, (c) to act in the best interests of patients are abridged by two conjunctive factors: (1) a valid advance directive or competent preference; and (2) the presence of an irreversible terminal illness. The factors themselves stem from vigorous bioethics debates about principles and axioms surrounding such matters as informed consent, the best interests of persons, personal identity, the validity of past or present decisions about future events, competency, advance directives, and the distinction between ordinary and extraordinary means.

The conjunctive factors may, in fact, be seen as rules for interpreting and weighting a set of principles in the clinical setting. Looked at in this way, the reasoning leading to the policy might look like 4j, 4k, and 4l.

In this example, the rules do not interpret the applicability of a moral principle to a situation, as they might in application-model or mediation-model reasoning. Instead they are used to adjust the relative importance of two moral principles in the design of a discretionary policy. We think the policy is still flawed because it does not address a third axiom -- the right to refuse treatment in situations other than terminal illness -- and also because it rests on an assumption that the distinction between ordinary and extraordinary means is still valid when deciding treatment options for the dying patient. We will have occasion to address the ruling of the New Jersey Supreme Court on the Conroy case in the next chapter -- a decision that dismissed the validity of the distinction in favor of a calculus of benefits and burdens.

For the moment, it is sufficient to note that policies are not formed only by deduction from several principles, political compromise, and weighting through rules. They are also validated and adjusted through implementation and consequent experience. Once general compromises and weightings have become standard practices, the emphasis of moral debate focuses on technologies that might fall under the policy. And this emphasis leads to a different focus of moral concern. This new focus then leads back to alterations in policy. The manner in which the use of intravenous fluids and nutrition has now come to be equated with questions about the removal of a respirator is a case in point, then, which has required further adjustment in the AMA policy, especially in its last assertion that when patients are not

4j

Major moral
principle: A physician's duty is to respect the right of patient self-determination while acting in the patient's best interests.

Descriptive factor: But in practice autonomy and beneficence often clash.

Normative
conclusion: A physician's duty is to "manage" properly the conflict between autonomy and beneficence.

4k

Normative premise: A physician's duty is to manage properly the conflict between autonomy and beneficence in caring for patients.

Descriptive factor: But proper management requires weighting these principles and constituent values differently in different situations.

Policy conclusion: A physician needs weights for the values of patient autonomy and beneficence specific to the situation.

4l

Policy premise: A physician needs weights for the values of autonomy and beneficence specific to the situation.

Rule premise: But
RULE 1: Autonomy takes precedence over beneficence when dying patients are competent, or if they expressed definite wishes applicable to this situation when they were competent;

RULE 2: Beneficence takes precedence over autonomy when irreversible terminal illness is not documented.
[Note: The AMA does not address in this specific policy patients who are not suspected of dying. It is not clear whether it accepts the right of all patients to refuse treatment noted by Veatch in argument 4a.]

Practical conclusion: 1. Advance directives and competent refusal of therapy when patients are dying are to be given precedence over a physician's duty to act in the best interests of patients.

2. If patients do not suffer from an irreversible terminal illness, physicians may continue to treat aggressively on the grounds of beneficence.

clearly dying, physicians are justified in aggressive treatment. This adjustment occurred in the March 1986 Judicial Council statement on fluids and nutrition.[44]

(15) The reason for this adjustment is that the case of Mr. Herbert in California (when two physicians were indicted for murder for removing IV fluids from a comatose but not brain-dead patient) marked the first time that an appellate bench equated discontinuing IV fluids (which before had been considered ordinary means) with removal of a respirator. The moral language shifted from categories of ordinary and extraordinary means to a language of proportionate and disproportionate care. This shift marked a transfer of emphasis "from the technique employed to the condition of the patient," as Paris and Reardon so succinctly put it.[45] Attention to hopeless but not necessarily "terminal" conditions such as dependent senility then occurred in the Conroy case,[46] the case of Mary Hier,[47] and the case of Nancy Ellen Jobes.[48] In the latter, as in the former, the court rejected the argument that nutrition should be distinguished from medical treatment, at least when it is delivered medically (through a nasogastric feeding tube in the Conroy case; through surgical implantation of a feeding tube in the stomach in the Hier case). Further, persons who are senile and debilitated, while not in common understanding terminal, were in effect considered as "dying patients" by the courts because the treatment at issue is to be measured on the basis of a benefit-to-burden calculus based on the patient's condition.

All of these changes in case law happened within two years, evoking the worst fears of those who see dominoes falling at every turn. And yet the logical progression in policy was inevitable once it had been established that neither patient autonomy nor physician beneficence (interpreted paternalistically) were absolute moral principles. Both had to be weighted and balanced against rules based on clinical parameters. The theory of a balance of principles continued to be validated in this way.

In this section, we have noted two sorts of validation models. In the first, represented by argument 4a, the application of theory differs only in degree from the mediation model in chapter 3. The difference lies in the use made of the descriptive realm, clinical data and practices, and legal precedents and decisions in validating an ethical theory embodying a single principle. The second set of examples demonstrated the ways in which an ethical theory of respecting a number of principles rather than just one leads to policies which are then tested and adjusted further, in which rules are used to weight the principles differently according to different clinical situations. Clearly, practice and experience are required to hone properly both the policies and the rules. We showed how policy about treating defective newborns resulted from extensive debate and clinical experience, and how it needed further modification. The same held true for the AMA policy on decisions dying people made about their care.

(16) There is yet another method of adjustment proposed by Terrence Ackerman.[49] Ackerman holds that the goal of bioethics is to reach policy or decisions which respect a maximal set of values and principles in a case. This is done by denying that there are any overriding principles in bioethics, just as Childress has now come to see. Ackerman's is a paradigm validation-model position. Indeed, he adds to the model a more scientific cast than the examples we have seen thus far. He proposes that experiments be conducted to determine whether or not the proper balance of principles has been achieved. The criterion of a justified policy is that it "effectively achieves the body of aims which persons involved would choose with adequate knowledge of the situation or set of situations in question."[50] The aims in any given case may or may not include a major moral principle. Since the experiment would be done on the effectiveness of the policy or decision based on what informed persons would choose as an outcome, it could be designed scientifically to measure whether the outcome was achieved.

It is clearer to us how this might be done for a clinical decision which respected a number of values of the (relatively few) participants involved, compared with a national policy. In the former instance, feedback could be obtained through a scientifically designed questionnaire, say, for cancer patients one is treating by balancing respect for their wishes and family decisions about burdens. In the latter instance, presumably an "Ackerman Test" could be designed to ascertain whether the Baby Doe rules struck the right balance. But in that instance, the polar dangers arise of (a) a fallout of responses along the lines drawn through the several years of bitter, acrimonious debate, or else (b) a policy distorted to the point of vacuousness in attempt to gain agreement among disparate parties.[51] Policies reached by political compromise may be a different kind than those reached by weights established by rules for which there is a high degree of consensus.

B. Strengths of the Validation Model

The strengths of the validation model are almost immediately obvious. First, this model has a healthy respect for the descriptive realm. While it still remains heavily deductive, it generally does not regard any single principle as sacrosanct. Hence its conclusions have the potential for appealing to a broader constituency than models which do not question fundamental ethical theory or a standard moral principle.

Second, because the model has a potential for widespread appeal, it can bear the burden of articulating and establishing public policy without totally abandoning medical and ethical values for others more pragmatic in tone, such as cost-effectiveness or public utility. A purely economic resolution of the challenge of treating defective newborns would look quite different from the Baby Doe rules. Cost-effective use of expensive interventions would be highlighted. As it is, no mention is made of economic values in the current law (except in connection with the penalty to states for failure to develop procedures for protecting infants from medical neglect). Instead the setting of limits to treatment is assumed under the ethic of not giving futile therapy.

Third, validation-model reasoning pays close attention to descriptive disciplines such as jurisprudence, sociology, psychology, legal decisions, medical anthropology, and the clinical practice of medicine itself. Recall that, in introducing the matter of this chapter, we spoke of clinicians' reactions to deductive ethics in application-model and mediation-model modes. Both have an element of unreality about them because the normative force stems entirely from apparently a priori principles. In the validation model that is not the case. The realities of life and of medical care receive some weight in the design of the policy. Thus they have a role to play, as filtered through the descriptive disciplines, with the very validation of the ethical theory.

Fourth, then, validation provides some inductive checks to unbridled deductive reasoning without falling prey to the naturalistic fallacy as Moore enunciated it.[52] The ethics of the action (except perhaps in Ackerman's view) does not stem from "what is." Yet "what is" helps determine the priorities of rank among principles which still carry the major part of the normative force of an argument.

Fifth, validation provides a kind of pragmatism, an action orientation, which forces theorists to pay more attention to the real-world consequences of reasoning about ethics. For many years ethics was dominated by meta-ethical concerns. By incorporating such matters as clinical practice, proportionality judgments of professionals, and the like into policies, the tragedies and victories of real human beings enter into our concerns for principled action.

Finally, it provides a method of reconciling conflicting moral principles in a policy. For example, autonomy and beneficence in examples 4j, 4k, and 4l are reconciled in application to treatment of the elderly through two moral rules, each reflecting a different clinical situation. Normally, proponents of each theory see an irreconcilable conflict between them. Recall examples 2g and 2h dealing with application-model reasoning (i.e., Sally Gadow's argument that the aged are best able to determine their own best interests with regard to health care). Gadow seems to misidentify beneficence with paternalism in her argument because she is so deeply committed to the principle of autonomy.   According to her position, the two principles could not be reconciled.[53]

D. Weaknesses of the Validation Model

First, while not as severe as in some of the models to follow, validation reasoning is subject to cautions about the naturalistic fallacy.   Such a fallacy often begins with quite reasonable inductive processes. In this regard, it is important to recognize the role of facts in establishing rules for judging which principle more validly applies to a given situation from a clutch of invaluable principles.   But in more extreme examples of validation-model reasoning, it appears that facts and data are used to validate principles themselves, since, as we have defined them, they are theoretical statements embodying experience and from which action-guiding statements can be drawn.

Second, from the point of view of ethics as principled action, the position depends overly much on policy consensus and nonmorally validated ends for putting principles into action. The answer to this objection is twofold, but each part is not without its own problems. First it might be said that validation-model reasoning does not validate principles so much as the *application* of principles to specific fields of activity as we said above. However, a strong form of validation-model reasoning (say Terrence Ackerman's proposal to verify outcomes through experiments) does seem to most observers to validate principles as well. Thus, as Marc Basson saw, Ackerman's proposal closely parallels medical decision-making.   Principles are simply summaries of previous bioethical decisions, rather than theoretical moral statements.   Basson's view is that Ackerman's account fails because it allows for no higher order standard of reference against which conflicting ethical intuitions may be judged.[54]   Basson argues that the proper method of such appeal is to appeal to the normative force of principles.   Ackerman's response depends upon a notion of "filling in," or altering moral principles.

This notion is derived from Richard Brandt's "qualified attitude method" as explained in his 1959 book *Ethical Theory*.   According to Brandt, principles in new situations must be altered, even if they have presumptive force: "Principles as we have them in mind must often be filled in, specified, or somehow supplemented."[55]   As Ackerman rightly notes, appeal to principles to resolve conflicting values simply cannot work, since there is no agreement in principle, and second -- and more problematically -- principles themselves carry no inherent or implied guidelines for prioritizing second-order principles and values implicit in different concrete situations.[56] (This point is also made above, in our critiques of the application and mediation models of reasoning.)   Hence, it seems clear that the validation model does, indeed, sometimes validate principles, not just their application to specific circumstances, even though it seems to consider principles themselves as nothing more than the embodiment of past experience. Consequently at least some forms of validation-model reasoning deny the prescriptive nature of moral principles which requires that principles *by definition* are applicable. Either moral principles are nonprescriptive (thus negating our modified definition of them), or this objection to the "Ackerman Test" holds.

A second way to answer the second objection is to indicate that nonmorally validated ends are not necessarily as dangerous in validation-model reasoning as they are to principled action from a position of cultural relativism. We shall argue in chapter 8 that the medical enterprise has an inherent moral character. If it is true, as we argue, that healing is a morally validated end, and the policies formulated in validation-model reasoning aim at that end in practice, then at least some of the force of the second objection is softened.

A final objection stems from concerns about rule by experts in modern society.[57] Some caution must be exercised about rule by experts to which this position is subject. Just as urban renewal policies developed by experts fell afoul of the profound values of neighborhood life in our large cities in the 1960s, so too will bioethical policies if developed only from ethical principles held dear by a "moral expert," or developed to defend only one morally "expert" point of view. This point applies also to the role of ethics consultations in hospitals.[58] The best way to ensure that rule by experts does not overtake validation-model reasoning is to incorporate all principles and viewpoints possible in the policy. But then, are we not back to Ackerman's view and its attendant problems?

Notes

1. These have been conveniently compiled into a volume, *Cases in Bioethics*, ed. Carol Levine and Robert M. Veatch (Hastings-on-Hudson, NY: The Hastings Center, 1983).

2. Terrence F. Ackerman, "What Bioethics Should Be," *Journal of Medicine and Philosophy* 5, no. 3 (September 1980), 263.

3. Ibid., 270.

4. Ibid., 260.

5. These conflicts occur on the micro-, macro-, and meso-levels, and they occur between and within patients, physicians, institutions, and cultures. See Jurrit Bergsma and Raymond Duff, "A Model for Examining Values and Decision Making in the Patient-Doctor Relationship," *Pharos* 43 (Summer 1980), 7-12.

6. Richard A. McCormick, *Health and Medicine in the Catholic Tradition: Tradition in Transition* in the Health/Medicine and the Faith Traditions series, ed. Martin E. Marty and Kenneth L. Vaux (New York: Crossroad, 1988), p. 5.

7. Ibid., p. 4.

8. Joseph Fletcher, "Humanism and Theism in Biomedical Ethics," *Perspectives in Biology and Medicine* vol. 31, no. 1 (Autumn 1987), p. 106.

9. Ibid, pp. 106-107.

10. Richard Selzer, *Confessions of a Knife* (New York: Morrow Books, 1987).

11. Consider the flap created by the publication of an anonymous story of a young resident who reportedly provided twenty milligrams of morphine to a twenty-year-old woman dying of ovarian cancer: "It's Over, Debbie," *Journal of the American Medical Association* 259, no. 2 (8 January 1988), 272.

12. For the initial Federal guidelines establishing IRBs, see U.S. Department of Health, Education, and Welfare, "Protection of Human Subjects: Proposed Policy," *Federal Register* 39, no. 165 (23 August 1974), 30648-30657. Current guidelines are contained in *The Code of Federal Regulations* 45 CFR 46 (Revised as of March 8, 1983).

13. *Bioethics Reporter*, Bioethics Subject File: "Hospital Ethics Committees: Laying the Groundwork" (January 1985).

14. American Academy of Pediatrics, "Guidelines for Infant Bioethics Committees" (1984). Unpublished document, available from American Academy of Pediatrics, 1300 N. 17th Street, Arlington, VA 22209.

15. David C. Thomasma and Joel Brumlik, "Ethical Issues in the Treatment of Patients with a Remitting Vegetative State," *American Journal of Medicine* 77 (August 1984), 373-377.

16. American Neurological Association, "Revised Statement Regarding Methods for Determining that the Brain is Dead," *Transactions of the American Neurological Association* 102 (1977), 192-193.

17. American Hospital Association, "Guidelines: Hospital Committees on Biomedical Ethics" (Chicago: American Hospital Association, 1984).

18.   American Medical Association Council on Scientific Affairs, "*In Utero* Fetal Surgery: Resolution 73 (I-81)," *Journal of the American Medical Association* 250, no. 11 (16 September 1983), 1443-1444.

19.   American Heart Association Committee on Ethics, "Ethics of Biomedical Technology Transfer," *Circulation* 67, no. 4 (1983), 942A-946A.

20.   American College of Obstetricians and Gynecologists, "Ethical Issues in Surrogate Motherhood," 1983 policy statement available from American College of Obstetricians and Gynecologists; 600 Maryland Ave., S.W.; Suite 300 East; Washington, DC   20024.   American Fertility Society ad hoc Committee on Artificial Insemination, "Report of Ad Hoc Committee on Artificial Insemination,"   1980 guidelines available from American Fertility Society; 2131 Magnolia Avenue; Suite 201; Birmingham, AL   35256.

21.   President's Commission for the Study of Ethical Problems in Medicine and Biomedical and Behavioral Research, *Deciding to Forego Life-Sustaining Treatment: Ethical, Medical, and Legal Issues in Treatment Decisions* (Washington, DC: U.S. Government Printing Office, 1983), pp. 248-249.

22.   Alasdair MacIntyre, *Secularisation and Moral Change* (Oxford: Oxford University Press, 1967), pp. 48-49.

23.   Daniel Callahan, "Shattuck Lecture: Contemporary Biomedical Ethics," *New England Journal of Medicine* 302, no. 22 (29 May 1980), 1228-1233.

24.   Arthur J. Dyck, "Ethics and Medicine," in *Ethics in Medicine: Historical Perspectives and Contemporary Concerns* ed. Stanley Joel Reiser, Arthur J. Dyck, and William J. Curran (Cambridge, MA: MIT Press, 1977), pp. 114-122, see especially pp. 119-120.

25.   Arthur J. Dyck, *On Human Care*, p. 20.

26.   Robert M. Veatch, *Death, Dying, and the Biological Revolution* (New Haven: Yale University Press, 1978).

27. The Society for the Right to Die (250 W. 57th Street, New York, NY 10107) has assembled a list of current resolutions of court cases involving the right of privacy and self-determination: Society for the Right to Die, "Right to Die Court Decisions" (New York: Society for the Right to Die, 1986). They have also assembled *Handbook of Living Will Laws, 1981-1984* (New York: Society for the Right to Die, 1984).

28.   G. R. Dunstan, "Ethical Aspects of Donor Insemination," *Journal of Medical Ethics* 1 (1975), 42.

29.   Carson Strong, J. S. Schinfeld, "The Single Woman and Artificial Insemination by Donor," *Journal of Reproductive Medicine* 29, no. 5 (May 1984), 293-299.

30.   U.S. Congress, Senate, "A Bill to Extend and Revise the Provisions of the Child Abuse Prevention and Treatment Act and the Child Abuse Prevention and Treatment and Adoption Reform Act of 1978, Amendments of 1983," S.1003, 98th Congress, 1st session; by Senator Jeremiah Denton (7 April 1983).

31.   U.S. Congress, House, "Child Abuse Amendments of 1984," Conference Report 98-1038. (Washington, DC: U.S. Government Printing Office; 19 September 1984).

32.   John C. Roberts and Donald H. J. Hermann, Untitled editorial in the *Chicago Tribune* (9 August 1987), Section 4, 2.

33.   Karen M. Forsythe, "Bill Protects Acts of Conscience," *Chicago Tribune* 25 August 1987, Section 1, 14.

34.   James F. Childress, *Priorities in Biomedical Ethics* (Philadelphia: Westminster Press, 1981).

35.   James F. Childress, "Ensuring Care, Respect, and Fairness for the Elderly," *Hastings Center Report* 14 (October 1984), 27-31.

36.   Cf. Norman Daniels, "Am I My Parents' Keeper?" in President's Commission for the Study of Ethical Problems in Medicine and Biomedical and Behavioral Research, *Securing Access to Health Care* (Washington, DC: U.S. Government Printing Office, 1983), Vol. 2, pp. 265-291.

37.   U.S. Office of Technology Assessment, *Life-Sustaining Technologies and the Elderly* (Washington, DC: U.S. Government Printing Office, 1987).

38.   This is the position of Norman Daniels, in *Just Health Care* (New York: Cambridge University Press, 1985).

39.   Mark Siegler, "Should Age Be a Criterion in Health Care?" *Hastings Center Report* 14 (October 1984), 24-27.

40.   Guido Calabresi and Phillip Bobbitt, *Tragic Choices* (New York: W. W. Norton and Co., 1978).

41.   Centers for Disease Control, "Prevention of Acquired Immunodeficiency Syndrome (AIDS): Report of Inter-Agency Recommendations," *Morbidity and Mortality Weekly Report* 32 (1983), 101-103; "Recommendations for Preventing Transmission of Infection with Human T-Lymphotrophic Virus Type III/ Lymphadenopathy-Associated Virus During Invasive Procedures," *Morbidity and Mortality Weekly Report* 35 (1986), 237-242; *Recommendations and Additional Guidelines for HIV Antibody Counseling and Testing in the Prevention of HIV Infection and AIDS* (Atlanta, GA: U.S. Department of Health and Human Services, Public Health Service, 1987); "Update: Human Immunodeficiency Virus Infections in Health-Care Workers Exposed to Blood of Infected Patients," *Morbidity and Mortality Weekly Report* 36 (22 May 1987), 285-289; *Guidelines for AIDS Prevention Programs, Operations* (Atlanta, GA: U.S. Department of Health and Human Services, Public Health Service, October 1987); "Recommendations for Prevention of HIV Transmission in Health-Care Settings," *Morbidity and Mortality Weekly Report* 36, no. 2S (21 August 1987).

42.   The American Hospital Association has appointed an *ad hoc* committee which is currently working out guidelines on this issue, as part of the work of the AHA Biomedical Ethics Advisory Committee.

43.   "Reports of the Judicial Council of the American Medical Association -- Dec. 1984," *Journal of the American Medical Association* 253 (26 April 1985), 2424-2425.

44.   Ibid., 2424.

45.   John J. Paris, F. E. Reardon, "Court Responses to Withholding or Withdrawing Artificial Nutrition and Fluids," *Journal of the American Medical Association* 253 (19 April 1985), 2243-2245.

46.   *In the Matter of Claire Conroy* 486 A.2d 1209 (1985).

47.   *In re Mary Hier*, Massachusetts Appeals Court, 4 June 1984.

48.   *In re Nancy Ellen Jobes* 108 N.J. 394, 529 A.2d 434 (1987).

49.   Terrence F. Ackerman, "Medical Ethics -- Its Role in Medical Care," *Forum on Medicine* 3 (July 1980), 448-449.

50.   Terrence F. Ackerman, "What Bioethics Should Be," 260.

51. Thomas Murray suggests that the latter was the result in the 1984 version of the "Baby Doe Rules"; see Thomas H. Murray, "The Final, Anticlimactic Rule on Baby Doe," *Hastings Center Report* 15, no. 3 (June 1985), 5-9.

52. G. E. Moore, *Principia Ethica.*

53. But see Edmund D. Pellegrino, and David C. Thomasma, *For the Patient's Good*, in which the authors argue that beneficence can incorporate autonomy through a concept of beneficence-in-trust.

54. Marc Basson: "Bioethical Decision-Making: A Reply to Ackerman," *Journal of Medicine and Philosophy* 8 (May 1983), 181-185.

55. Richard Brandt, *Ethical Theory* (Englewood Cliffs, NJ: Prentice-Hall, 1959), p. 247.

56. Terrence F. Ackerman, "Experimentalism in Bioethics Research," *Journal of Medicine and Philosophy* 8 (May 1983), 169-180.

57. Robert M. Veatch, "The Medical Ethicist as Agent for the Patient," in *Clinical Medical Ethics*, ed. Ackerman et al., pp. 59-67; Peter Singer, "Moral Experts," *Analysis* 32 (1972), 115-117; Stephen Toulmin, "The Tyranny of Principles," *Hastings Center Report* 11 (1981), 31-39.

58. Kai Nielsen, "On the Need for 'Moral Experts': A Test Case for Practical Ethics," *International Journal of Applied Philosophy* 2, no. 1 (Spring 1984), 69-73.

CHAPTER FIVE
The Determination Model

A step further towards giving primacy to practice rather than to validation or alteration of prior principles is one in which some version of practice *determines* moral theory. This is clearly a more inductive moral reasoning process, since it proceeds from categories of practice to the establishment of moral theory. In this approach, between practice and policy formation is inserted some further set of factors which arises from contexts of practice and *determines* either the ethical theory to be employed or the set of principles which will predominate in the decision of a course of action.

To see where this model stands in relation to others we have sketched, let us review the path we have taken thus far. In the purely deductive model, the conclusion is entailed in the premises, the normative principles, to such an extent that no further determinations are admitted. As we move towardsever more inductive models, the middle premise becomes less and less descriptive. Interpreting this premise requires a set of moral rules. In the more deductive models of this move, the moral rule is singular (or, if we begin with more than one moral principle -- as in Ross's system -- and conflict develops, then one set of rules is ultimately given primacy over the others). In the validation model outlined in the preceding chapter, the moral rules are plural, thus leading to policies which attempt to protect several principles at once. The most extreme form was one in which the principles are validated on the basis of experiment or experience with the consequences of a policy directly formulated to respect a maximal set of values and principles.

In clinical-context reasoning, the medical context itself functions as the moral rule. Thus the context can determine which theory, principles, or axioms ought to predominate in the resolution of cases. To some extent, by determining the principles which are germane to the case at hand, the context actually determines the principles which flow from it (to speak properly, since they are not "applied to" the situation). The reason this is so is that, by definition, principles must apply. If the context, functioning as a moral rule, determines that some principle is not germane, then that principle fails to "apply" to the case and its nonrelevance may be said to have been determined by the rule. That is why we call clinical-context reasoning the determination model.

The clinical-context reasoning model is different from the approach taken by Ackerman that was discussed in the previous chapter. Determination here takes place by appeal to *categories of practice*, some distinct form of practice, rather than by appeal to *experiment* or experience with consequences, for example, to determine what one should do. The determination model is also different from the origination model (to be examined in the next chapter). In origination-model reasoning, one moves inductively from the case at hand to pick and choose values to be respected in the case. The *existential case* itself functions as the context, as the moral rule interpreting the process and content of the resolution attempt.

An example will help to make this difference clear. A decision to honor the wishes of a dying alcoholic to receive no special therapy (e.g., blood transfusion) to prolong his life when his liver fails, could be made on several distinct grounds and in several distinct contexts. The first might be that of the primary-care context in which a physician has built up a long-term care relationship.[1]   Within the context of that relationship, the physician agrees that his patient's wishes ought to be respected, especially since there are no other countervailing circumstances or interests. Even if treatments were available that offered a significant prospect of prolonging life, the physician would give considerable weight to the patient's reluctance to undertake them.

A second, alternative, reason might be entirely different. The alcoholic makes his request in an intensive-care unit after his liver has failed. He is severely bloated, and is bleeding from the esophagus as well. The physicians (who may have little, if any, past knowledge of this patient's thinking on matters of life and death) consider a number of values and eventually agree not to prolong his life on the grounds that, in their *experience*, any further efforts ultimately prove fruitless in this sort of case and the alcoholic eventually dies anyway. They hold that the best way to approach the clinical management of end-stage alcoholism is to honor the wishes of patients not to be treated. If patients request aggressive treatment, they comply -- but with a sense of tragedy, futility, and economic injustice.

A third method for making a decision in this case would be to treat each case entirely on an individual and personal basis. This latter is a form of situation ethics which will be discussed in the next chapter.[2]

In the first example, the principle of respect for persons is presupposed in the decision to respect the patient's wishes. This principle is determined to apply to the case through the axiom of autonomy because of the *context* of the primary care relationship. The physician's past dealings with this patient have stressed negotiations which attempted to help the patient ascertain his wishes in regard to the medical matter at hand and then to accommodate those wishes insofar as this physician's personal and professional conscience allows. In the second example, the principle of respect for persons is balanced with a number of other principles -- such as not prolonging dying, cost-effective humane care, the prolongation of life, and the patient's autonomy; and the principle of respect is chosen or "validated" for the case on the basis of *experience* (or clinical experiment) in which it has been revealed that the outcome for such patients is better served if one respects patient wishes to forego treatment.

In short, validation reasoning explored in the previous chapter looks to consequences through policy formation to help validate moral theory. The form of determination reasoning -- the matter for this chapter -- is less consequentialist. Instead, the context in which medicine is practiced determines which theories shall emerge or predominate. The applicability of a given theory depends upon the context in which it is employed. The contexts themselves interpret the principles and theories and their relevance to the case.

Clearly some appeal to context is always necessary to interpret principles and to determine their applicability to matters at hand. The minor premise of the practical syllogism in application-model reasoning consists of a description of (selected) elements of the context of action. But determination-model reasoning gives greater weight to context than this simple appeal. Normally, ethicists regard the appeal to context as guided by moral principles or rules after the fashion we have already discussed in chapters 2, 3, and 4. The categorical imperative might be invoked to interpret the principle of autonomy by commanding some form of action by which that principle is protected. Or the "principle" (actually, moral rule) of the double effect might be discussed as a justification of giving a dying patient sufficient morphine to control distress and yet recognizing that this would have the undesired (but not necessarily unwelcome) effect of killing him, due to depressed respiratory sufficiency -- thus interpreting a way of doing good in a certain situation without intending evil.

In this chapter, by contrast, we will examine the ways in which the medical context itself functions as a moral rule, aiding the resolution of medical ethics quandaries. We will first examine the moral rules which can help determine the appropriate moral theory, and then, as in previous chapters, discuss the strengths and weaknesses of this mode of reasoning.

A. Context and Moral Rules

(1) A middle course between a generalist application of ethical theory and specialized case-by-case analysis is possible with a contextual grid for medical ethics advanced by one of us (Thomasma).[3] It is only one example of work on contexts to which medical ethics must address itself. Neither axioms nor standard moral rules are sufficient (although they are necessary, of course) to determine the validity of moral theory and ethical principles in resolving medical ethics problems. Additional rules, or guidelines for relating theory and practice, must be developed according to this approach. Among these rules is the context functioning as a formal adjustment to values in concrete circumstances.

The root of the difficulty in medical ethics lies in a confrontation between an abstracting tendency in the long and rewarding history of ethics and the concrete, individual problems encountered by professionals. The latter must make quick decisions about very complex matters in order to benefit their patients. Contrariwise, ethical analysis must take careful note of numerous ethical theories, axioms, and other concerns in order to conduct a minimally decent conceptual and problematical analysis. This process takes time and, of necessity, becomes quite abstract. Health professionals and patients quickly lose interest in these abstractions and theoretical meanderings if they are not decisively and explicitly related to the realities of patient care. They must do ethics on the run.

Ethical principles appear abstract -- or better, speculative -- because they do not possess the same degree of social legitimacy as the values of everyday life. Moral abstractions frequently are seen by nonphilosophers as empty of the normal ingredients of moral concerns people have in their day-to-day life. No doubt they can and do seep into that daily life, but the process of connecting theory to practice is a long and subtle one in most cases. Thus, according to the "contextual grid" theory, what is needed is a means by which to locate a moral problem and to exhibit the likely values and principles at issue within that locus. The context having been established by such a "grid," the discussion can proceed towardsmeans for resolving the case by protecting the interests and values of those affected by it.

There is a variability of contexts in the clinical resolution of cases that is noticeable to all who work in the medical setting. This variability does not describe so much the relativity of values and principles; rather, it describes how the weight they bring to bear on a case is partially determined by the medical specialty involved; the personal values of the patient, family, or social group; the personal and professional values of the health care professionals involved; and the institutional setting in which the problem arises. Some principles and axioms will be given more weight than others in such a scheme, and one important component of the weighting will stem from the contexts.

Such a contextual grid is only one component, then, of what might be called context-variable moral rules. Other examples we examine in this chapter do not fit the contextual-grid pattern, but are moral rules which in other ways vary with the context. Further, the contextual grid Thomasma proposes cannot encompass all of the variables in a case -- but only the ones most likely to be affecting the emphasis of some values or principles over others. (Recall the weaknesses of the deductive models in this regard.) As we saw, the rule of protection of autonomy is more likely to be given prominent focus in a primary-care context than in a tertiary-care one, wherein one's autonomy is virtually always depressed and thus concern for autonomy is diminished in favor of a goal of preservation of life and/or restoration of health.[4] Furthermore, the rule of protection of autonomy is more likely to be emphasized in cases in which there is no threat to others than in cases wherein the common good must be considered, sometimes to the detriment of personal autonomy. Finally, because the grid only *describes* most likely weights given to moral principles and rules in formulating an indicated course of action, one should not misconstrue the contextual grid as claiming that physicians in tertiary-care settings do not care about protecting their patients' autonomy, or that public health officials stress social responsibility to the exclusion of individual well-being. All of these moral values bear upon a case. The grid only describes what values are most likely to take precedence over others.

The contextual grid theory rests on two distinctions. The first is the distinction between primary-, secondary-, and tertiary-care settings, a standard distinction in medicine. This distinction forms one set of coordinates of the grid. Its importance for moral reasoning lies in the seriousness of the assault on personal wholeness brought about by the disease in question.[5] Thus, a patient's wishes are more likely to be sought and respected in a primary-care setting than in an emergency room after a heart attack, where a paternalistic response may be, and often is, more appropriate. The second distinction or coordinate of the grid is that between the individual and the number of persons affected by the problem. The moral significance of this distinction is based on the increasing complexity of values the more different persons whose interests are affected by the outcome of the case enter our consideration, and our increased tendency to protect the commonweal the greater the number of affected persons. Recall again the purpose of the grid is to describe context-variable rules, which principles and axioms in any particular moral theory are likely to be given more weight than others in a given circumstance in formulating a moral policy or in developing an indicated course of action.

The grid is illustrated in figure 3.

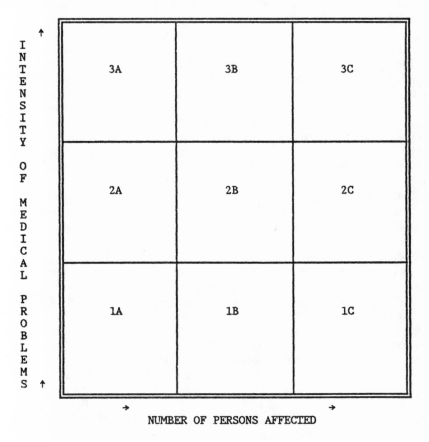

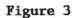

Figure 3

1. Definitions

1. In figure 3, quadrant 1a represents a single doctor-patient relationship in a primary-care nonserious or only mildly serious situation, 1b represents the same situation also affecting a family group, and 1c the same situation affecting the larger society in some way. A good example to illustrate these different categories might be a mild infection. Suppose 1a represents a throat infection easily cured with an antibiotic. No problem. But suppose 1b is a highly contagious disease. The patient's personal concerns may have to be modified somewhat in the interest of protecting his or her family from the disease. Quadrant 1c might be a venereal disease, such as gonorrhea. Here the patient's values must now be meshed with social concerns about reporting that disease, and thereby checking the spread of this infection across society.[6] As noted in chapter 4, AIDS reflects just such a social concern. Because of its potential for destroying the lives of others, even on level one (before it fulminates into a tertiary care requirement), AIDS falls into quadrant 1c.

2. Quadrants 2 represent a serious, single medical problem which can be reversed, while a, b, and c stand for (respectively) individual, family, and social interests in the case. A good example might be a heart attack. In 2a, the patient is recovering from the acute attack in a ward room, and her wishes and concerns can be primary. In 2b, the focus is on long-term recovery, which now must be meshed with family values which might have contributed to the pressures leading to the heart attack in the first place. Autonomy is circumscribed by health concerns. The president of a university may have to step down, or suppose the patient has a history of alcohol ingestion and smoking, but these she identifies as "crutches" to help her cope with an unfaithful husband. Concerns about her recovery, and her desires, must now be placed within the context of the family. In 2c, her recovery will necessitate care in a nursing home. This outcome means that her grandchildren may have to sacrifice buying a new car in order to help place her there, and her own home may have to go on the market. Her shop, where she exchanged paperback books, may have to be closed -- which will have an impact within the whole community in which it is located.

3. Quadrants 3a, 3b, and 3c represent parallel outcomes, but now for a life-threatening event. In 3a, a man is brought to the emergency room, the victim of an automobile accident. He is unconscious and has sustained massive brain damage. His own values are of less concern at this moment than saving his life. Even if he were a Jehovah's Witness, the tendency would not be to respect his right to refuse blood on the face of it. In 3b, a family is trapped in a burning home, and the firemen might have to decide which person to rescue in a situation in which it is unlikely that all can be saved. The worst

case for individuals is 3c, in which a life-threatening event affects society itself. A good example was the control of the bubonic plague in Italy. If one member of the family contracted it, the entire family was boarded up in the home, and the house burned (killing all the occupants). The common good clearly was seen as taking precedence over individual merit or rights. The Chernobyl disaster is another example. A huge population was re-settled in another part of the Ukraine to minimize the disastrous effects of radiation exposure.

2. Single Example

Another way of illustrating the grid is through a single example. Take population ethics.

1a: An unmarried adult requests sterilization. The request is not medically indicated. The patient's right of self-determination is the primary value to be preserved because there are no other interests in the case.[7]

1b: A married adult requests sterilization. The request is not medically indicated. However, family obligations and economic factors demonstrate a reasonable cause. The patient's right of self-determination must be balanced with the physician's obligation to do no harm and the current values of the family.

1c: A married adult requests sterilization. The request is not medically indicated. Further, the married partner objects and, for religious reasons, hospital policy does not permit sterilization. Since more social involvement occurs in this quadrant, social values and institutional norms may sometimes predominate. The patient may have to go elsewhere to receive what he or she wants.

2a: A married patient with a chronic illness requests sterilization, without which a pregnancy may threaten her life. She is a diabetic on renal dialysis. Thus, the sterilization is medically indicated. Both the principles of self-determination and beneficence require the sterilization, but the risks of the operation on the chronic illness must be weighed and perhaps other methods of contraception explored.

2b: A severely retarded adult, unmarried, is considered a candidate for sterilization by her family prior to being placed in a large home for retarded children. Her family's desires, however, must be integrated with laws protecting the retarded and the retarded child's own wishes, if ascertainable.

2c: A moderately retarded child is sexually active and parents request sterilization. However, society's own eugenic laws, the interests of the retarded as a class, and the individual determinations of judges and health professionals may override the personal preferences in this case.

3a: A married, pregnant woman, contracts leukemia, necessitating a therapeutic abortion to allow radiation and chemotherapy. Note that while the individual rights of patients are horizontally preferred in the grid and in quadrant 3, these must be balanced against the factors of serious disease. Another example of 3a concerns might be a D & C after a rape, even though the individual would desire to have children if conceived in a loving relationship. Most often quadrant-3 cases are crises which appear in emergency rooms and intensive care units, in which the values of the patient are hard to obtain, and individual rights are protected only insofar as there are presumptions for a value of continued life.

3b: A nuclear accident occurs in which five women employees and their fetuses are exposed to damaging amounts of radiation. Despite individual values in normal circumstances, the level-3 intensity of the danger of this exposure to their lives and to their fetuses might require termination of their pregnancies.

3c: In this quadrant, the classic case of enforced sterilization of a population in a poor country can be placed. Individual rights and family rights are superseded in favor of economic development. Suffice it to say that such social programs rarely work!

What is important to note about the single-case example is that absolute moral prohibitions rarely, if ever, apply. Sterilization is not always morally wrong; neither is abortion from the point of view of contextual analysis.

3. Context and Moral Rule

Note that instead of deriving a syllogism to illustrate the grid, we have been forced to describe a number of cases whose outcomes may differ precisely because of the context. It is possible, however, to list the ways in which the context of practice does function as a moral rule, using the grid as a formal, contentless example:

1a. Horizontal: The further one moves to the right, the less important individual rights become, and the more is valued the axiom of beneficence. Similarly, the principles of the common good and the greatest happiness take precedence over the patient's individual rights. Bear in mind that the grid presents only a means by which to clarify the context and the most likely principles and rules in conflict. It may provide a means by which to resolve the conflicts, but it is not directly a normative guideline for a course of action. More about this point in a moment.

Second, the further one moves across the horizontal axis, the less the personal responsibility of the physician is emphasized, and the more weight is given to health professionals' social responsibility. This is another way of stating that the common good, for example, in controlling health-care costs, must enter the weighting of values the physician and patient consider in their negotiations.[8]

1b. Vertical: 1, 2, and 3 represent the clinical contexts of medical care: primary, secondary, and tertiary care. Primary care deals with front-line, noninvasive, preventive, and basic care for nonserious or only mildly serious problems. In this context even considered horizontally, the patient and his or her values take precedence over all other values, with corresponding horizontal diminishment. In secondary settings, mostly hospitals, nursing homes, and chronic disease settings, less of the patient's own values and more of the contex's predominate.   In tertiary-care situations, other individual values are sacrificed for the fundamental value of preserving life, or horizontally, preserving society itself.

This descriptive grid can be helpful as a corrective to single-principle ethical resolutions, which neglect the clinical context of medicine. Prolongation of life, for example, is a substantially different problem in quadrant 1 than in quadrant 3. In 1, a healthy patient may have a seizure in a doctor's office and intervention is warranted; in 3, this may be the fourth seizure in a day -- each leaving the patient more and more a vegetable -- and intervention may not be warranted. The obligation to preserve life is different in 2 than in 3c, when a physician may have to choose from among a number of persons severely injured in an earthquake.   Thus, any attempt to discuss medical ethics problems without attention to these significantly different quadrants or contexts at best provides only a polemic for one's moral principle or its refinement, and at worst demonstrates an insensitivity to concrete moral quandaries which would render the discussion fruitless.

But is the contextual grid merely descriptive, as has been claimed? Does it provide no more than a description of the balances and priorities among principles and axioms commonly struck in suggesting a policy or course of action? Can it have any normative force on the outcome of a decision? If it were merely descriptive, then it would have no impact on the problem of justification of indicated courses of action by appeal either to absolute moral principles, intermediate axioms, or moral policies. The grid should be seen as a suggestion about how one might appropriately rank such morally important factors in specific contexts.

A major problem in understanding how to justify particular ethical recommendations or an indicated course of action is that "intermediate principles" or axioms conflict in specific circumstances. (This was a weakness of the mediation model.) Indeed, in some cases moral principles themselves come into conflict, as we have seen in previous reasoning models. The task of medical ethics must therefore be to set priorities among conflicting values. One method of setting the priorities is, not by appeal to external moral justifications (as in the mediation model) or by appeal to respecting several moral rules at once in a policy (as in validation-model reasoning), but rather by appeal to the context of action.

The context itself suggests how the priorities should be arranged. An emergency room is not a place for developing the sort of professional-patient relationship that gives primacy to patient's wishes. The physical structure of the facility, staffing patterns, the form of records storage, and the nature of conditions characteristically seen all preclude leisurely, in-depth exploration of personal values and dictate instead a focus on the immediate medical problem. The morally significant question may be, not should patient autonomy be given primary focus in emergency rooms, but rather should we *have* emergency rooms or, instead, organize all medical care in private-practice primary-care structures. The growth of freestanding acute-care treatment centers may indicate a preference by some patients for this style of care over traditional primary-care approaches. This process of analyzing the context is nonetheless a descriptive process. In fact, it might even be called a circumscriptive process, since placing a person within a quadrant on the grid involves both descriptive, factual material and circumscriptive attention to other possible locations on the grid.

The validity of this approach depends upon descriptive validity. The moral arguments center on the appropriateness of *location*.

(2) Abstracting from the contextual grid proposed by Thomasma, what does determination reasoning look like when encountered in the usual medical ethics literature? Let us examine the New Jersey Supreme Court disposition of a well-known case, that of Claire C. Conroy,[9] to note how transferring persons among categories of practice changes the moral character of the arguments in their regard. In the Conroy case, there is a descriptive definition of dying which, in effect, moves Ms. Conroy from the category of "old, debilitated, and senile" to the category of "irreversibly, terminally ill." As McCormick indicates, "My own opinion on these issues is that permanently comatose and *some* noncomatose but elderly incompetent patients may be classified broadly as dying."[10] As a consequence of this move to another context, the usual principles applying to the dying are then applied to her situation. In other words, by interpreting Ms. Conroy's situation under the new category of dying, a context shift has taken place, not unlike reclassifying a patient on the Thomasma grid from level 2 to level 3. With that shift come new responsibilities and considerations. No longer is prolonging life a primary or overriding moral duty. Instead the overriding moral duty is now not to prolong dying (especially if the process is painful).[11]

Claire Conroy was an old woman who could no longer feed herself, or accept feeding by others. The nursing home taking care of her wanted to insert a nasogastric feeding tube into her nose through to her stomach in order to feed her. Her nephew objected. The nursing home prevailed, but he chose to go to court to argue on his aunt's behalf, since he was the only surviving near relative and was already designated her legal guardian. This case reached the Supreme Court of New Jersey which issued its ruling after Claire Conroy had died with the feeding tube in place.

The court set out three rules on the basis of which one can withdraw life-prolonging therapy from such patients. The preference, of course, lies with obtaining the wishes of the patient; and thus for competent patients this is the determining factor. But, as the court maintained, the right to reject treatment remains intact despite the level of the patient's competence. If the patient does become incompetent, as was Claire Conroy, then a surrogate decision maker acts on the patient's behalf. In light of this overriding consideration, treatment most often would be withheld or withdrawn on the basis of presumed prior wishes, if no explicit wishes are known. It would not be based on the social worth of the patient, the value of the patient's life to others, what reasonable persons might wish in a similar circumstance (the "reasonable persons" test), or even what other, competent patients have chosen to do in similar circumstances.[12]

The tests proposed by the court are summations of current ethical and legal thinking about respecting the autonomy and decision-making capacities of patients, and, in their absence, appealing to the best interests of such patients, as far as possible determining such best interests on the basis of presumed wishes and medical indications. The tests are listed below in order of preference. One starts with the first test. If that cannot be used, then one moves to the second, and finally to the third.

Test 1, The Subjective Test:
Life-sustaining treatment can be withheld or withdrawn from an incompetent person when it is clear that the person would have refused treatment under the circumstances.

A surrogate decision maker would, at this point with test 1, appeal to past decisions the patient made to argue the case that the patient would clearly not want this treatment now. The appeal cannot rest on quality-of-life judgments or the reasonable-person criterion, however. Rather it is made on the basis of "clear and convincing evidence" about the patient's prior wishes -- such as a "Living Will" or other advance directive documents[13] they have executed, or explicit statements they made to family, friends, or health professionals. Presumably the patient's value history would be relevant here, as McCullough and Beauchamp pointed out.[14]

The latter two tests are used when the patient has left no explicit statement about preferences, nor exhibited behavior which would form convincing indication of their wishes in the present situation.

> *Test 2, The Limited Objective Test:*
> Withholding or withdrawing treatment may also occur if there exists some trustworthy evidence of the person's preferences *and* the substitute decision maker determines that the burdens of continued life with the treatment in question outweigh the benefits of continuing that life.

This test or rule may also be called the Best Interest Test Number One because it combines a preference-component (based upon "trustworthy evidence") with a benefits/burdens calculus. Note that the benefit and burden are not calculated on the basis of impact on others, but rather on the impact on the life the patient now lives. Just as in the 1958 address by Pope Pius XII to anesthesiologists on the use of the respirator, the focus of the moral discussion lies on the treatment.[15] Is the treatment burdensome? Does the treatment make only a marginal difference in the existence of the person? Is the person's quality of life enhanced by the treatment?[16] The quality of life judgment made in this test, and in the next one, is not a utilitarian judgment. Instead, it is based on the bodily impact of the treatment and its outcome. It employs the language of proportionality instead of categorical determinations of ordinary or extraordinary means.[17] Thus, proportionality of treatment to outcome for the patient's quality of life becomes an overriding consideration once the patient is moved from the category of "alive but weak" to "dying."

> *Test 3, Pure Objective Test:*
> Lacking any presumed wishes or any trustworthy evidence of patient preferences, one may still withhold or withdraw treatment on the basis of medical indications, proportionality, and cruelty. The net burden of the treatment in question must be judged by the surrogate decision maker to clearly and markedly outweigh the benefits the patient derives from life. Further, the pain associated with the treatment must be judged disproportionate to the impact of the treatment on the patient's condition such that to instigate the treatment or to continue it would constitute cruelty or inhumaneness.

This test may be called the Best Interest Test Number 2, since the surrogate must still make a judgment about what would benefit the patient, even in the absence of good evidence about what the patient would want. Since the judgment about outcomes in this instance is almost entirely based on objective data, the court called it the "pure objective" test, although it hardly is purely "objective" in the ordinary sense of that term.

In fact, we would have preferred for the Court to recognize the concert of interests involved in treating the patient at this stage. The care givers should also have a say in the treatment of the patient in this circumstance, since they often have a better grasp of the data and potential impact of the treatment. At the heart of the ruling is a second context-determination: a judgment that food and water, if delivered by medical means, can be forms of medical care, and are therefore subject to the same constraints as other medical interventions.

It now would be revealing to try to construct an inductive form of the arguments in the Conroy case. They might appear as shown in 5a.

5a

Indicated course
of action: Physicians may withdraw or withhold life-prolonging treatment
                    from patient X, who is now incompetent.

Moral policy: Supporting this action is a moral policy stating at least:
                    1. That feeding by IV lines and through a nasogastric
                    feeding tube is a medical, not just a symbolic, procedure.

(Supporting this element of the policy are court decisions to consider feeding through medical interventions as medical procedures subject to the same moral considerations as high-technology interventions such as respirators.[18] The court decisions, in turn, were based upon the arguments of a group of philosophers and physicians who, abandoning the distinction between ordinary and extraordinary means as a normative category, claimed that food and water can unduly prolong life as much as higher technologies.[19] Courts have explicitly rejected the notion that IV fluids and nutrition have a symbolic value that ought to be respected, as Callahan has argued.[20])

---

                    2. Discontinuance of feeding through medical
                    interventions need not involve aiming at the death of the
                    patient.

(Supporting this element of the policy is the traditional distinction of the double effect.[21] By withdrawing such treatment one intends a kindness, not the death of the patient, which must come about indirectly. To discontinue the treatment in order to bring about the death of the patient is to will directly that the patient die, and may constitute a form of euthanasia bordering on active. Although scholars are divided about the double-effect rule,[22] it is nevertheless clear from the Conroy case tests that the proper judgment for withholding and withdrawing is the patient's best interests; and quality of life, not bringing about the patient's death. Not considered by the court, apparently, is the notion that sometimes death itself may be a kindness and a "benefit" to the patient.)

---

3.   The burdens/benefits calculus includes a quality-of-life judgment.

(Supporting the ingredient of the policy is a frank admission of quality-of-life judgments in such cases. Although the court seemed to try to avoid such judgments, they are unavoidable as soon as appeal is made to the benefits/burdens calculus. Recall, however, that this judgment is made about the benefits *of the treatment* on the patient's existence, not the life itself. Thus, the judgment must be drawn at the right place.[23]   As the court indicated, one cannot make the judgment for economic reasons or on the basis of merit, or the value of the patient's life for another.)

Moral rule: The context will determine the extent to which the quality-of-life judgment will be valid. In general, a weak, debilitated, incompetent, senile patient may be considered to be dying.

Principles: 1. All patients, even comatose or senile or otherwise incapacitated persons, preserve the right to refuse treatment.
                              2. The duty of professionals towardsthe dying is not to unduly prolong their dying.
                              3. The value of human life is not absolute.
                              4. It is the quality of human life, not just its biological existence, that makes life worth living.

By spelling out the argument as an inductive process, one can more clearly detect the ways in which the context of care, and the decision about the extent of criticality of the patient *determines* the moral weight given to the principles which buttress both the policy and the indicated course of action. A category of practice, treatment of a nursing-home patient, has altered or determined our moral theory about how to approach that patient. The nasogastric feeding tube is judged too "outrageous," too disproportionate to the quality of life the patient enjoys in her bed, to benefit her in any real way. It merely prolongs what is now judged to be her irreversible, terminal illness-- senile old age.

(3) Another example of determination-model reasoning, in which practice determines the moral theory to be applied in cases, comes from the reflections of Eric Cassell, a physician who frequently writes on philosophical issues. For many years, he has opposed the notion that there is a single moral principle in medicine, especially if that principle is to be seen as autonomy.[24] Struck by Hartshorne's notion that life is a work of art, he was prompted to argue that rules about autonomy and overriding autonomy, tests of the right to self-determination, and tests of the right for physicians' paternalism seem, from the perspective of aesthetics, to be "ugly." He claims instead that complex values can be ordered aesthetically, beyond considerations of paternalism and autonomy. This ordering might take place in a kind of life-world, a larger context in which life itself and its deeper values relativize the usual and excessive concern about autonomy and paternalism.   In this regard, Cassell argues that autonomy is particularly inappropriate as a fundamental principle because it rests on a view of persons as discrete, separate, isolated entities. He says:

> What is necessary is a wider set of values in which medicine serves the purposes of sick persons. In that larger framework, concepts like autonomy serve a more useful function by promoting an understanding of the place each person has in creating the texture and design of her or his own life.[25]

The idea of creating "texture and design" is what prompts attention to the aesthetic elements of this broader moral theory, in which autonomy and other principles find a place. The broader moral theory itself is urged on us by the experience of a clinician. Cassell finds something "ugly" or wrongheaded about the rules and regulations surrounding current cases, such as that of Elizabeth Bouvia, who asked a hospital in California to help her die. She was quadriplegic and could not help herself out of a life she regarded as difficult and useless.

It would be tempting to argue that Cassell has erred through a category confusion between art and morality; and aesthetic judgment of one's life is not the same as ethical analysis of it. Yet his insight does provide grounds for reexamination of an ethic which proceeds by principles alone, as the application and mediation models do, for example. The corrective he offers is that there is a larger life context that establishes the moral character of a person's life, in which various moral principles are chosen depending on the circumstances. As such, then, his is a determination-model approach.

The inductive reasoning would appear as shown in 5b.

5b

Indicated course of action:	Patient Sam Smith should be treated in light of his value history.
Moral policy governing the course of action:	Individuals in medical care should be treated according to a complex of values rather than a set of principles imposed from outside the doctor-patient relationship. This complex of values should include the individual's own value history as revealed in the relation between doctor and patient.
Context functioning as a moral rule:	Life is an extremely rich, almost aesthetic experience, in which individuals carve out their own value framework. This complexity is revealed in the clinical setting in a way that is inaccessible to ethical theories that stress principled reasoning processes.
Principles:	Autonomy of the patient. Beneficence of the physician.

Note that Cassell does not argue that any one principle would predominate depending on the context, as one might in the contextual grid model. Rather, Cassell wishes to stress the individuality of the decisions to be made without intrusion by a vortex of public rules and regulations. In this, his proposal is closely related to one we will examine in the next chapter proposed by Stephen Toulmin. Nonetheless, it is still a model in which the context, in this case the life-world of the patient, determines the normative theory to be applied to that patient, that is, a theory which balances different ethical principles with the value history of the patient. We have taken liberties with his notion of life as a work of art by substituting the value-history concept of Beauchamp and McCullough for the idea of individuals creating the "texture and design" of their own lives, in order to avoid a potentially distracting discussion of aesthetics and ethics.

(4) In more general terms, the contexts of medicine function as moral rules. They assist in the application and relative balancing of values in cases, rather than as interpretations of the meaning of principles themselves. This insight can clarify a number of problems raised about competing methodologies in medical ethics and the role of the realities of clinical practice in deciding which method is more meritorious as an aid to medical decisions. Some readers might have wondered with us, for example, how it was possible that Beauchamp and Childress, who adopt opposing moral theories could, from their separate principles, arrive at concurring conclusions.[26] We asked whether principles matter at all in designing ethically justified courses of action? One answer to this problem lies in the nature of middle-level axioms and rules. Interpretation through such axioms and rules of relatively contentless principles may quite easily lead to similar conclusions, especially if the axioms arise from the practice of medicine itself and the moral rules occur in the medical context.

A second possible answer to the problem of the role of principles is that contexts, functioning as moral rules, provide the means by which a number of principles or values are combined to bring about a resolution of the case. Unlike the situation cited in the previous paragraph, in which principles are given content by axioms and then applied in context, this second scenario represents a change in deductive methodology itself. Instead of application of a single principle, such as the principle of autonomy, a number are joined together in context to protect as many values in the case as possible. In this approach to the problem of moral principles, their absoluteness is denied (since a number of competing principles are given equal weight), but their worth or relevance to the case is upheld.

A third possible answer to the problem of moral principles is, of course, that they do not matter at all. Responding to Thomasma's argument that the autonomy model for the doctor-patient relation is limited,[27] Dr. Zawacki[28] suggested a resolution of the autonomy-beneficence quandary through negotiation between doctor and patient at the bedside. This negotiation is not unlike a suggestion elsewhere, that both the doctor's and patient's conscience must provide a discretionary ethics to resolve the inadequacies of autonomy or paternalistic models.[29] Nonetheless, this inductive position cannot be left to subjective relativism alone. As Howard Brody puts it: "Some guidelines for conscience must prevail in the process."[30] At this point, in order to escape relativism and subjectivism, the context can function as a mold in which similar cases can be examined by a process of analogical reasoning, a type of contextual grid.[31]

In each of these methodological patterns, the context functions as a moral rule, providing guidelines either for the *application* of principles (in a deductive model), the *joining* of principles (in a casuistic model), or the *induction* of analogues (in a nonsubjectivist inductive model).   To be sure, there are quite a few other methodological models available in medical ethics. But these three suffice to indicate how it can be understood that a context could function as a moral rule.

(5) Before turning to our final example -- from Paul Ramsey's writings -- we should note that arguments about the moral status of the fetus in the abortion debate can often take the form of the context determining moral theory. Think of how the arguments progress from the biological life of the fetus (i.e., whether it is a person, or simply an animal life-form) to its claims on the values of the mother and on society. If the fetus is declared to be a person or potential person, the argument's context becomes one in which conflicting personal rights (i.e., fetus and mother) are argued and debated. One must choose which is more important, the right to life of the fetus or the mother's right to privacy (i.e., to make her own decisions about what would happen to her body). If the fetus is declared to be a "lump of flesh," a "growth," or an "appendage" of the mother's body (positions which are less defensible today in light of modern fetal science than they were even ten years ago), the debate's context moves from conflicting rights of persons to the mother's personal and social responsibility.[32]

(6) By briefly alluding to the abortion debate, we move from models in which the context merely *describes* which principles will predominate in practice (at best a sort of quasi-normative process without real normative force) to a model in which the context *determines* the ethics of an action itself. We think Paul Ramsey's "medical indications" policy from his book *Ethics at the Edges of Life*[33] fits into the latter category. He discusses the issue of abortion and problems of ethical judgments for dying patients (those at the edges of life), including seriously ill newborns. In order to avoid any hints of quality-of-life judgments (as later the *Conroy* court failed to avoid them), Ramsey in effect edges out all remnants of moral principles in making judgments for dying patients -- appealing instead to medical indications alone. Recall the "pure objective" test discussed earlier in connection with *Conroy*. In that test, one makes a benefits/burdens judgment regarding the life of the patient and the treatment in question, *coupled* with this question: Does this treatment stand up to a medically indicated course of action? If so, it must be given. If not, it is optional.

As a backdrop to his study of medical indications, Ramsey is concerned that in decisions to be made, equity is to be preserved. Thus, he frequently discusses *categories* of cases that would not receive treatment. For example, categories of children who would not be treated if defective, or categories of persons who would not receive open heart surgery (e.g., all stroke victims) are described. To do otherwise than to make decisions in terms of such categorizations would be to fail to acknowledge the "equal and independent value of human lives."[34]

But how are the categories to be chosen? The principle of selectivity for treatment, if it is not to be based on social worth or other quality-of-life-tinged rules, would have to be an objective categorization or classification of patients, determined not by their merit or the value of their lives, but wholly by the nature and extent of their disease. And that is where the "medical indications" policy comes in. One determines treatment plans on the basis of clinical judgments about diseases and accidents -- actually the only purely objective basis we possess.

Although Ramsey employs the policy throughout his book, he develops it most fully for making decisions about dying patients. He argues that there are really only four standards for making decisions to withhold or withdraw treatment: the ordinary versus extraordinary means distinction; the standard medical care policy; a patient's right to refuse treatment; and a medical indications policy. He then proposes a reductionist defense of his approach: "I shall argue that the significant moral meaning of these similar and related standards can be reduced almost without significant remainder to a medical indications policy."[35]

The way this is done is to point out that the standard medical care policy in which one compares various appropriate treatments is always relative to the patient's own present condition, not some abstract notion of a standard of care to be given. Quality of life judgments are inappropriate because they would impose an external valuation on the merit of an individual's life. Further, the patient's right to refuse treatment is not absolute:

> Why not say that the classification "ordinary/extraordinary" can simply be reduced to (1) a determination either of the treatment indicated or that there is no treatment indicated in the case of the dying, and (2) a patient's right to refuse treatment? The answer to that question is that there are medically indicated treatments (these used to be called "ordinary") that a competent conscious patient has no moral right to refuse, just as no one has a moral right deliberately to ruin his health. Treatment refusal is a relative right, contrary to what is believed today by those who would reduce medical ethics to patient autonomy and a "right to die."[36]

Having thus reduced all of the other standards for withholding or withdrawing care to what is medically indicated, he is left with the "medical indications policy." According to this policy, treatments are given or withheld on the basis of treatment that is indicated:

a medical indications policy that readily allows for treatment indicated or no further curative treatment indicated in the case of the dying . . . . It directs attention to the objective condition of the patient, *not* to abstract classifications of treatment or to the wishes of any of the parties concerned -- not even to the previously expressed opinion (as reported) of Karen Ann Quinlan.[37]

We are now able to see what Paul Ramsey has accomplished in the medical indications policy. Perhaps without intending to, but rather intending to eliminate quality of life and patient autonomy considerations, he has actually eliminated all extraneous matter from ethics (if that is the correct way of speaking)! The inductive argument might appear as shown in syllogism 5c. Note that the principles hover around in the background, but actually do not enter the medical indication judgments, and therefore have no normative force in the action to be performed.

5c

Indicated course of action:
> James Smith, who is dying, will be treated objectively according to what is medically indicated by his condition.

Medical indications policy:
> All dying patients shall be treated according to objective medical indications required by their condition (including, in some cases, no treatment at all).

Context as moral rule:
> The patient's condition determines the treatment to be offered.

Axioms which determine the policy:
> There is no absolute right to refuse treatment.
> Quality-of-life judgments are to be avoided.
> Some treatments are not optional, especially if they can save
>   life.

Principles (hovering about but not having a direct impact on either the policy or the indicated course of action):
> All persons must be treated fairly and equitably.
> Human life must also express higher values than life itself.
> Personal intersubjectivity, relationship with God and others, is
>   the highest principle of life.

Unlike the other examples, then, in which the context functions to determine which principles shall predominate in the course of a treatment, either by using a grid, or through the judgments of physicians about the value history of the patient, or even the patient's own condition (as in the *Conroy* tests), Ramsey's medical indication policy *itself* determines the moral theory. It *is* the moral theory. It is an objective standard by which to determine which treatments should be employed.

Ramsey himself attempts to sum up the conclusion he has reached in a curious footnote, which we attempt to amplify in the presentation below. Following each of his statements, we have added an expansion of it -- filling in his number-reference by the relevant statement.[38]

If this is the content of the "medical indications" policy, it is certainly no improvement over other proposals in terms of clarity. We leave it to the reader to ascertain whether this set of principles forms a coherent and satisfactory policy for decision-making in life-and-death cases. What this approach clearly does *not* do, however, is to reduce decisions to an objective "medical indications" standard as Ramsey promised. None of the five distinctions drawn at the outset consists wholly of medical indications. The distinction between 2a and 2b comes closest to this, although physicians report difficulties making a firm classification of patients in these terms. 3a and 4a may be medical categories, but the notions from which they are distinguished (i.e., 3b and 4b) are clearly extramedical. And, the contrasts drawn in 1 and 5 are commonsense conceptual points, not technical judgments of medicine. Given these features of the constituent concepts, we cannot expect the axioms set out in Ramsey's footnote to incorporate wholly *medical* indications.

B. Strengths of the Determination Model

The determination model shares many of the same strengths and weaknesses as the validation model.

Its first strength is its clinical compatibility. As we mentioned in the Introduction, the practice of medicine is inherently important for ethical decision-making. Because the determination model focuses so well on the context, and from it, derives moral meaning, it can provide such meaning for the patient and doctor in the gradual unfolding of the clinical event.

Second, like the models to follow, it respects the clinical contexts in which the meanings arise. As we saw, the contexts themselves provide moral weights for making decisions. Since the most critical function of ethical decision-making in the practical realm, the realm underlined by Dewey and Tufts in our frontispiece, is precisely the weights to be given to different values embodied in principles, axioms,

. . . wrong-making is now one of the consequences of continued appeal to the distinction between ordinary and extraordinary means as mere classifications, . . . [i.e.] when the class meaning of extraordinary (or morally dispensable) means is used by someone who fails to distinguish
  1) between a) conscious decision to refuse treatment in one's own case, *and* b) withholding treatment in the case of another;
  2) between a) "terminal" patients who are dying, *and* b) "terminal" patients who are simply incurable;
  3) between a) medical help, *and* b) prolonging dying;
  4) between a) biological indices for medical help, *and* b) socioeconomic measures of burden or advantage to come for the primary patient; *or*
  5) between a) medical help for a primary patient, *and* b) relieving the burden or serving the advantage of others.[17]

NOTE 17: The following tabulation might be made of some of the conclusions suggested by the foregoing chapters.

If 3a and 4a are the case, 1b is not morally permissible for 2b, 4b or 5b reasons;

> **If 3a** [medical help may be effective] **and 4a** [there exist biological indices for medical help], **then 1b** [withholding treatment in the case of another] **is not morally permissible for reasons of 2b** ["terminal" patients who are simply incurable], **or 4b** [socioeconomic measures of burden or advantage to come for the primary patient], **or 5b** [relieving the burden or serving the advantage of others].

1a may be morally permissible or even praiseworthy for 2b, 4b or 5b reasons even if 3a and 4a are the case;

> **1a** [conscious decision to refuse treatment in one's own case] **may be morally permissible or even praiseworthy for reasons of 2b** ["terminal" patients who are simply incurable], **or 4b** [socioeconomic measures of burden or advantage to come for the primary patient], **or 5b** [relieving the burden or serving the advantage of others], **even if it is the case that 3a** [medical help may be effective] **and 4a** [there exist biological indices for medical help].

1b is morally permissible if 2a;

> **1b** [withholding treatment in the case of another] **is morally permissible for 2a** ["terminal" patients who are dying]

2b patients, given that 1a is not the case, should be evaluated for treatment in terms of 4a and 5a and the availability of 3a;

> **2b** ["terminal" patients who are simply incurable], **given that it is not the case that they have made any 1a** [conscious decision to refuse treatment in their own case], **should be evaluated for treatment in terms of 4a** [biological indices for medical help], **and 5a** [medical help for a primary patient] **and the availability of 3a** [medical help]

1b is morally permissible even if 4a is the case, if there is no 3a or if to attempt 3a would likely do more harm;

> **1b** [withholding treatment in the case of another] **is morally permissible even if 4a** [there exist biological indices for medical help] **if there is no 3a** [medical help], **or if to attempt 3a** [medical help] **would likely do more harm**

1a is morally permissible if 2a.

> **1a** [conscious decision to refuse treatment in one's own case] **is morally permissible for 2a** ["terminal" patients who are dying].

professional conduct, institutions, cultures, and previous moral choices made by the principals in the case, the determination model offers more than the validation model in this regard.

Yet, as a third strength, it shares with the validation model a place for ethical principles, unlike its more inductive cousin, the origination model (to be explored in the next chapter). Granted, the principles have now lost some of their power of entailment. One cannot deduce conclusions directly from them. Yet they still influence (not govern) the outcomes of decisions in the concrete realm in this model.

Perhaps the most important strength of the determination model is that it provides explicit (and therefore arguable) means for prioritizing middle-level axioms, rules, and ultimate principles. By this is meant that the explicit criteria, often unexamined in more deductive models, can be subjected to debate, and themselves critiqued and refined. This is important for the negotiation about values that must take place in the doctor-patient relation, as we shall argue in constructing a unified theory of clinical ethics in the final chapter.

C. Weaknesses of the Determination Model

The danger of the naturalistic fallacy looms even larger in the determination model than it did in the validation model. Much of what was discussed there need not be repeated here. Are we to assume that moral meaning that does arise from specific contexts will determine the outcome of decisions, as the principles and axioms of ethics stand by only to "lend a hand"? This appears, on the face of it, to vitiate the power of principles and place too much trust in the practical affairs of human life, its structured (and culturally determined) organization. Yet it is important to note that the fundamental assumption of the determination model is that those structures, indeed, contain codices of the good, from which ethical decisions can be "read."

The second problem of the determination model is its loss of logical rigor. Compared with the first two deductive models, its forms of reasoning appear obtuse and overly complex. Precisely because no single principle is deemed prescriptive enough to command an action in the practical realm, the complexity of the world of action, and its supposed structures, make reasoning difficult.

Third, as mentioned above, there is a danger of reaching temporally or culturally determined and conditioned responses. Just as the Roman Catholic Church might argue against women priests (a current moral crisis) by appealing to its traditional practice-structures ("We have never had women priests." "Jesus was a man."), so too might reasoning from practical structures in medical ethics lead to equally culturally conditioned ethical decisions. A good example of this danger can be found in physician arguments for traditional medical paternalism: "I have found in my practice that patients really do not want to make decisions. They want the doctor to make them for them." Even though this may be, in fact, true, does the determination model require us to accept this experience as an embodiment of authentic moral values? Perhaps it is at this point that the respect for principles might help the model.

Yet, even though it does provide a place for principles and axioms, note that these have been relativized by the context. While not as contentless as in the origination model to follow, the principles' very application to the matter at hand depends upon the context (functioning as a moral rule, a moral interpretant). The best one can hope for in this model is an experience of the "rightness" of the decision based on a variety of goods, goods both hidden and explicit, in the structures, principles, and axioms. This "rightness" is always open to continued critique. If one keeps this openness to critique in mind, then the ethical decision is never a final one. The self-critical awareness of decisions reached in this model require a sense of unfinishedness to all ethical decisions. Unlike medicine that seeks a "clinical closure," there can be no "ethical closure," even when a decision is made.

Perhaps the most difficult problem the determination model faces is its technology-dependence. There is always a danger of reduction of the moral crisis to what is currently possible or in vogue in medicine. Recall how the contextual grid was organized according to current clinical practice: primary, secondary, and tertiary care. These distinctions can be artificial, especially if a patient falls between the categories. Further, they are heavily dependent upon the technological capacities of modern, Western medicine. A good example of these capacities can be gleaned from the liver transplant program. A person with a failed liver can be in a hepatic coma, and within a day after transplant, be awake and interact with his or her family and care givers. This is a sort of resurrection afforded by modern medicine. Lazarus is raised from a state of death. Yet because medicine is now committed to the person who has received a transplant, the context itself drives the moral rule that emerges when the first, second, and even the third transplant on that person has failed. The rule might be stated as follows: "The patient entered our hospital dying. She will either leave dead, or alive. We will not cease trying to save her until it is no longer possible." But the technology-dependent character of this rule, dependent as it is on the tertiary transplant care, neglects other important moral values. Among them might be the enormous cost of saving one life compared to providing access to health care for all. Another might be the "vampirization" of a city's blood supply (liver transplants take up to forty units of blood) to the detriment of

others. Still a third consideration might be the value of the place of
others on a waiting list for the scarce resource that is a liver, while
one uses up to four on a single person to whom one is already
committed.

These concerns require more than negotiation about values in the
doctor-patient relation. They require ongoing social discussion and a
search for consensus about important values in a community. Medical
ethics is only in the initial stages of this search.

NOTES

1. For an analysis of such a relationship, see Pellegrino and Thomasma, *A Philosophical Basis of Medical Practice*, especially chapter 10, pp. 223-240.

2. For a further list of considerations which might be given for terminating treatment, see Graber, Beasley, Eaddy, *Ethical Analysis of Clinical Medicine*, pp 184-185.

3. David C. Thomasma, "The Context as Moral Rule in Medical Ethics," *Journal of Bioethics* 5 (Spring/Summer 1984), 63-79.

4. David C. Thomasma, "Beyond Medical Paternalism and Patient Autonomy: A Model of Physician's Conscience for the Doctor-Patient Relationship," *Annals of Internal Medicine* 98 (1983), 243-248.

5. Jurrit Bergsma with David C. Thomasma, *Health Care: Its Psychosocial Dimensions* (Pittsburgh: Duquesne University Press, 1982).

6. Cf. Graber, Beasley, Eaddy, *Ethical Analysis of Clinical Medicine*, pp. 58-61, *et passim* 53-72.

7. Glenn C. Graber, "On Paternalism and Health Care," in *Contemporary Issues in Biomedical Ethics*, ed. John W. Davis, Barry Hoffmaster, and Sara Shorten, (Clifton, NJ: Humana Press, 1978), pp. 233-244.

8. E. Haavi Morreim, "Cost Containment: Issues of Moral Conflict and Justice for Physicians," *Theoretical Medicine* 6, no. 3 (October 1985), 257-279; see also E. Haavi Morreim, "The MD and the DRG," *Hastings Center Report* 15, no. 3 (June 1985), 30-38.

9. *In the Matter of Claire C. Conroy* 98 N.J. 321, 486 A.2d 1029 (17 January 1985).

10. Richard A. McCormick, "Caring or Starving? The Case of Claire Conroy," *America* 154 (6 April 1985), 269-273.

11. Paul Ramsey, *The Patient as Person*.

12. David C. Thomasma, "Ethical Judgments of Quality of Life in the Care of the Aged," *Journal of the American Geriatrics Society* 32 (July 1984), 525-527.

13. Chris Hackler, Ray Moseley (eds.), *Advance Directives* (New York: Praeger Press, forthcoming).

14. McCullough and Beauchamp.

15. Pius XII, "The Prolongation of Life," *The Pope Speaks* 4, no. 4 (1958), 393-398.

16. Joanne Lynn, "Brief and Appendix for *Amicus Curiae*," *Journal of the American Geriatrics Society* 32, no. 12 (1985), 915-922.

17. Benedict M. Ashley, OP, and Kevin D. O'Rourke, OP, *Health Care Ethics: A Theological Analysis*, 2nd ed. (Saint Louis: The Catholic Health Association of the United States, 1982).

18. Rebecca Dresser and E. B. Boisaubian, "Ethics, Law and Nutritional Support," *Archives of Internal Medicine* 145 (January 1985), 122-124.

19. Kenneth C. Micetich, Patricia H. Steinecker, David C. Thomasma, "Are Intravenous Fluids Morally Required for a Dying Patient?" *Archives of Internal Medicine* 143 (May 1983), 975-978; Joanne Lynn and James F. Childress, "Must Patients Always Be Given Food and Water?" *Hastings Center*

Report 13, no. 5 (October 1983), 17-21; Joanne Lynn (ed.), *By No Extraordinary Means: The Choice to Forego Life-Sustaining Food and Water* (Bloomington, IN: University of Indiana Press, 1986).

20. Daniel Callahan, "On Feeding the Dying," *Hastings Center Report* 13, no. 5 (October 1983), 22.

21. Austin Fagothey, *Right and Reason*, 6th ed. (Saint Louis: C. V. Mosby, 1976), pp. 32-33; Gerald Kelly, *Medico-Moral Problems* (Saint Louis: Catholic Hospital Association, 1958), p. 20; Richard A. McCormick, *Ambiguity in Moral Choice* (Milwaukee: Marquette University Press, 1973).

22. Philippa Foot, "The Problem of Abortion and the Doctrine of Double Effect," *Oxford Review* 5 (1967), 5-15; Glenn C. Graber, "Some Questions About Double Effect," *Ethics in Science and Medicine* 6 (1979), 65-84.

23. Richard A. McCormick, "Caring or Starving?"

24. Eric Cassell, *The Healer's Art* (New York: Lippincott, 1976).

25. Eric Cassell, "Life as a Work of Art," *Hastings Center Report* 14 (October 1984), 35-37.

26. Beauchamp and Childress, *Principles of Biomedical Ethics*.

27. David C. Thomasma, "Limitations of the Autonomy Model for the Doctor-Patient Relationship," *Pharos* 46 (1983), 2-5.

28. Bruce Zawacki, "Letter to the Editor: Limitations of the Autonomy Model," *Pharos* 46 (Summer 1983), 42-43.

29. David C. Thomasma, "Beyond Medical Paternalism and Patient Autonomy: A Model of Physician Conscience for the Physician-Patient Relationship," *Annals of Internal Medicine* 98 (1983), 243-248.

30. D. Brody, "The Patient's Role in Clinical Decision-Making," *Annals of Internal Medicine* 93 (1980), 718-722.

31. David C. Thomasma, "The Context as Moral Rule in Medical Ethics."

32. H. Tristram Engelhardt, Jr, "The Beginnings of Personhood: Philosophical Considerations," *Perkins Journal* 27, no. 1 (Fall 1973), 20-27.

33. Paul Ramsey, *Ethics at the Edges of Life: Medical and Legal Intersections* (New Haven: Yale University Press, 1978).

34. Ibid., p. 282.

35. Ibid., p. 155

36. Ibid., p. 156

37. Ibid., p. 159

38. Ibid., p. 330

CHAPTER SIX
The Origination Model

In chapter 5 we examined in detail ways in which an inductive model we called "determination" assisted resolution of medical ethics quandaries. The determination model did so by employing inductive reasoning based on categories of practice to establish the appropriateness of moral theory or principles, which were themselves embedded in the contexts of practice. The context also determined which theory or which principles ought to predominate in the move from policy formation to practice.

This chapter now examines an even more fundamentally inductive approach that we call the origination model. As we did in previous chapters we shall first describe examples of this model of reasoning, and then present its strengths and weaknesses.

Origination is a purely inductive model. From descriptions of states of affairs in medicine one is led to the development of axioms and further, to the development of a new moral theory itself. One does not make appeal to rules or categories of practice (as in the previous two models) to delineate or determine which preexisting theories or principles should weigh more heavily in the balance when moving from policy to action. Instead, the inductive process itself leads by inference to general or universal statements that are the product of induction. For this reason we call them inductive products or generalizations. The problem for this method of reasoning is to note from what source these statements acquire normative force. If there is no appeal to "outside" norms, then can descriptions of what is the case lead to ought statements?

A. Origination and Experiment

(1) The first example of the process illustrates the direct line taken in the inductive approach from states of affairs to inductive products without appeal to an "outside" norm. Recall at this point our definition of an axiom. This example also illustrates how purely inductive ethical reasoning parallels that of clinical judgment.

Over one hundred years ago H. Worthington Hooker became distressed by the problem of truth telling in medicine. He noted:

> Every day we see evidence of the fact that so large a proportion of the medical profession practice deception upon the sick, that the profession as a whole has to a greater or less degree the imputation fastened upon it.[1]

Hooker attacks the problem by reasoning from cases.[2]

This reasoning from experience leads him to a series of axioms governing the relationship of truth and deception in clinical affairs. The reasoning is sophisticated and finely tuned. One can catch a faint echo of Kant in one axiom ("If it be adopted by the community as a common rule, that the truth may be sacrificed in urgent cases, the very object of the deception will be defeated.")[3]; a hint of rule utilitarianism in another (". . . the good which may be done by deception in a *few* cases, is almost as nothing, compared with the evil which it does in *many* cases . . .")[4]; elements of pragmatism in still another ("If the deception be discovered or suspected, the effect upon the patient is much worse than a frank and full statement of the truth can produce.")[5]; and a concern for the virtues of trustworthiness and confidence, as well as truthfulness ("the *general* effect of deception, aside from the individual which it is supposed it will benefit, is injurious.").[6] Inductive reasoning, as we shall see in the next chapter, can rely on the virtues as interpretants of situations.

It is noteworthy about the inductive process of reasoning Hooker employs, and about the inductive process in general that the process of reasoning is:

1. *Case driven*. That is, a particular instance of some troublesome occurrence (in this case, the practice of deception) prompts the thinker or practitioner to examine the problem in more detail. Among cases he cites are that of a mother coaxing a child to take medicine, a friend not being told her friend has died, and so on.

2. *Eclectic*. That is, sources feeding the reasoning process come from many disciplines. Hooker cites, for example, a statement in Percival's *Medical Ethics* that details instances wherein one may "depart" from the truth. In particular, Percival permits lying to protect patients, a point Hooker finds objectionable, as we shall see. But the context of this section of his book makes it clear he has considered arguments from many sources.

3. *Analytically Diverse*. The generalizations (axioms or middle principles) appear to be identifiable parts of accepted larger theories, yet the thinker does not consider himself or herself committed to any one or another of these theories. Note at least four such statements in Hooker's analysis.

4. *Axiomatic*. Nonetheless, a general axiom is finally proposed -- what we call an inductive product, that arises from the case matter and the other sources. It is important to stress that the ethical process derives its moral weight from within rather than by appeal to external weighting factors (rules) or other theories. It appears almost as a "compromise from within," derived from the thinker's own considerations. His reasoning appears as shown in 6a.

6a	
Descriptive premise:	Considerable confusion among patients and in society is generated by the practice of lying to patients.
Inferential premise 1:	Such confusion is caused by a series of injuries or harms to the relation of confidence that ought to exist between doctor and patient, as well as harms to society itself.
Inferential premise 2:	These harms are pragmatic and ethical, destroying in turn the virtue of the physician, and the patient's and society's good.
Inferential premise 3:	Yet sometimes it is necessary to withhold a truth from patients which it is feared might be injurious to them.
Inductive Generalization:	"In withholding the truth no deception should be practiced, and that if sacrifice of the truth be the necessary price for obtaining the object, no such sacrifice should be made."

Hooker's conclusion[7] is clearly a compromise. It is not, however, a compromise between competing ethical theories like deontologism and utilitarianism. No theoretical debate or abstract priority principle is offered. Instead what is presented is an internal compromise, between the clinical necessity of not harming patients and the pragmatic and good moral consequences of truth telling, not only for patients, but for the profession as a whole, as well as for society.

(2) A good, modern example of the challenge of truth telling comes from a heart transplant program. As one patient described her experience, upon awaking from the anesthesia, she kept asking whose heart she had received. In part this desire to know was prompted by gratitude, and in part by simple curiosity. The transplant team would only tell her from which hospital it came and that the heart was over twenty-seven years old. She continued to press for more information. Being a nurse herself, in the end she recognized that "It was right not to tell me more. Now I don't feel as if I'm borrowing someone else's heart. It's really mine."[8] The transplant team did not lie to her, they just told her that they were not at liberty to divulge any more information. Withholding the truth did not involve a sacrifice of the truth. The team's concern for the healing process, which included the patient's taking ownership of the heart, was not compromised by injurious lying. Hooker's inductive generalization was employed to good effect.

(3) Contrast the heart transplant case with telling the truth to a spinal-cord injury patient. It is common practice in rehabilitation medicine to hold out therapeutic goals that the staff know ahead of time are unreasonable and unattainable. Thus an athletic teen, the victim of a diving accident, after ten days is completely paralyzed from

a spinal cord fracture at C-6 and C-7, and is incontinent of bowel and bladder.   Yet after four weeks, some recovery of movement and strength occurs in both arms.   His left lower extremity exhibits full passive range of motion but decreased active motion, with only 2-3/5 muscle strength.   His right lower extremity also shows full passive range of motion but virtually no active, due to only trace muscle movements and strength of only 0-1/5. Unable to walk or even keep his balance while seated, the patient is, however, highly motivated. He is told he might walk again with a lot of work, even though the staff are virtually certain this is impossible, because they want to maintain his optimism.

As Sissela Bok notes, lying may sometimes be justifiable if it can benefit the patient, but the burden of proof lies with the physician.[9] Beauchamp and Childress hold a somewhat similar position, namely that a wrong may be done to satisfy *prima facie* duties of "highly significant importance."[10]   Of course, the rehabilitation team has determined that the lie is justifiable because holding out optimism at this stage will help the patient gain whatever function he can (however little).   This is the duty of "highly significant importance." Note how an ethics derived from principles and duties draws balances between competing principles, duties, and values, and in this case, permits lies, however infrequently (in contrast to Hooker's position).

(4)   A more stringent position against lying to patients was developed by Richard Cabot, like Hooker a distinguished physician. Cabot determined to establish an experiment about truth telling rather than   engage   in   endless   debates   pitting   assertion   against counterassertion. Today we would find the experiment flawed due to low numbers of patients and failure to satisfy other sophisticated criteria of research methodology.   But Cabot was satisfied with the results of his eight years' observation. He decided to tell the truth to his patients and record what happened. This was in contrast to the practice of equivocation and lying he had learned earlier in medical school. He was particularly interested in whether there would be any untoward side effects.[11] Other physicians had argued, on an anecdotal basis, that real harm could come to patients if the truth were told them of their condition. One case concerned telling the wife of a patient with serious heart disease that he would die when the wife herself had serious heart trouble coupled with a proclivity to overreact.

Cabot's experiment covered diagnosis, prognosis and therapy. It revealed no difficulties with truth telling. In fact, many important benefits accrued from telling the truth. He noted: "I have not yet found any case in which a lie does not do more harm than good."[12] His argument could be summarized as shown in 6b, 6c, and 6d.

The first thing to note about this reasoning process[13] is that the generalization can lead directly to a policy about truth telling, and also

6b

Descriptive premise:	Ambivalence exists among doctors about telling patients and families the truth about their disease.
Inferential premise:	The ambivalence rests on a concern not to harm patients or families.
Inferential premise:	Harms ought to be measurable enough to be subject to experimentation.
Inductive Proposal:	An experiment rather than debate may prove which is the better course to take, telling or withholding the truth.

6c

Inductive proposal:	An experiment may prove which is the better course.
Procedural premise:	Patients and families will be told the truth about their disease.
Observed Result:	The results of telling the truth produced many benefits and fewer harms to patients than lying.

6d

Observed result:	The results of telling the truth produced many benefits and fewer harms to patients than lying.
Procedural premise:	Anyone can carefully duplicate these results.
Inductive Generalization:	"The technic of truth telling is sometimes difficult, perhaps more difficult than the technic of lying, but its results make it worth acquiring."

to practice in individual cases.   As we said, this inductive process parallels the formation of clinical judgments in some instances.   A physician begins her practice with a few notions.   Experience with a great number of cases leads her later to ponder what works best for a class of patients.   Following this a policy might be developed for the office.   This policy would lead directly to practices implementing the policy.   A good example might be that of a family physician's efforts to get psychosocial information about problem-oriented histories from patients.   Suppose this effort resulted from years of experience in trying to treat patients.   Eventually the physician settles on a policy of asking all patients to fill out a thorough questionnaire addressing these issues before being seen by the nurse and prepared for the physician encounter.

In a similar vein, Cabot's experiment proceeded towardsa conclusion that led to a policy of truth telling.   But where did it acquire its normative force?   It certainly did not acquire it from a deductive reasoning posture, in which the moral theory of respect for persons led to an axiom regarding truth telling, and a policy on this point.   And yet one gets the sense that such a theory and its norms function as a backdrop to the inductive process, even though no direct borrowing of an axiom is made to give the conclusion its normative force.

The reason that impression exists is that the concern about not harming patients is part of the inductive premises in all our examples so far.   This concern exists precisely because of a traditional Hippocratic imperative to help or at least to do no harm.   Yet this imperative (prescription if you will) does not function as a norm in the reasoning process.   Even so, it may be the key to answering how the inductive process can lead to an inductive generalization possessed with normative force.   At any rate, we shall discuss the role of "outside" normative influences on inferential ethics logic later in this chapter.

B. Negotiation

(1) Another example of a purely inductive process might come from the psychology of medicine.   Studies have been done on the impact of disease on persons.   In the last chapter we noted how Eric Cassell used this data to argue that philosophers of autonomy forget that people have bodies, and that the impact of disease on the body may impair autonomy.   Although he did not present the following argument, one could easily construct it from his reasoning as shown in 6e.[14]

In this example the scientifically observable impact of disease on persons leads to a specific axiom or policy about the care of the seriously ill.   As such it is an excellent example of Origination

6e	
Descriptive premise:	Disease has a major impact on the function of the body.
Inferential premise:	If one takes persons as a synthesis (self) of body and ego, disruption of the body has an impact on the ego and on self.
Inferential premise:	Autonomy involves self-determination and the authenticity of choice.
Inductive generalization:	Autonomy is impaired by disease.
Policy statement or axiom:	The special vulnerability of the sick must be respected.

reasoning. It is driven by the distress of disease to a moral category of humane and respectful care.

(2) A sixth example of purely inductive reasoning comes from Mark Siegler, also a physician. In this example Siegler enunciates a general view, almost a "situation ethics" of medical practice. In it, little is found of ethical theory (except as the view itself is an ethical theory). In fact, few axioms are enunciated either.

Guidance about decisions must be entrusted to morally conscientious physicians. Each clinical encounter is considered unique as is, consequently, the degree of autonomy the physician and patient wish to have. Patients and physicians therefore must accommodate to each other's values.[15] Siegler's description of the doctor-patient relation has subsequently come to be called the fiduciary model. But this description is usually accompanied by an appeal to a guiding principle of beneficence, rather than basing the relation wholly on negotiated values, as Siegler seems to do in his argument.[16]
Siegler's argument is capped by this paragraph:

> Moral and technical arrangements of each medical encounter are determined mutually, voluntarily, and autonomously by both physician and patient. Accommodation is a process of communication and negotiation, sometimes short and to the point, sometimes extended, as to what rights and responsibilities each participant wishes to retain and which will be relinquished in the context of their medical relation.[17]

Clearly, the model put forth by Siegler requires a dynamic, changing process of dialogue, in which both physician and patient contribute. Furthermore, both must possess certain virtues, like trustworthiness, fidelity, promise keeping, and respect for the autonomy of the other.

The methods of communication needed in this model are not spelled out, but openness, honesty, and reflexivity about values is assumed.

Siegler's inductive approach to moral certainty in medicine is mapped in 6f.

6f

Descriptive
Premise: The doctor-patient relation is the source of morality in medicine.

Inferential
Premise: Morality in medicine is derived from accommodations about values in that relation, especially values about duties and rights.

Inductive
Generalization: The axiom governing the doctor-patient relation ought to be that all values be negotiated.

Note how Siegler's reasoning is almost purely inductive. There are no specific rules or theories the doctor and patient must follow in developing their negotiated values. Howard Brody criticizes this extreme inductivism as follows:

> Medical situations differ in many respects, but also reveal striking similarities. Unless we can pull out some general principles as we go along, we will never be able to apply to new cases what we have learned from previous ones.[18]

Indeed, from Siegler's other writings, and from the context itself, one is aware of the nonmaleficence backdrop, namely that one must not harm the patient.

Extrapolating from Siegler's view to an even more general one regarding inductive argumentation from a single case, the reasoning might appear as shown in 6g.

Loretta Kopelman has tellingly pointed out the strengths and weaknesses of the "case studies" approach. In her view, the use of a case-studies approach in medical ethics can help solve a number of problems; in particular it can contribute to a rich and diverse approach to the realities of ethical dilemmas. A proper use of cases, too, can help correct the view that "moral rules [are] inherently derivative from particular decisions or cases."[19]   Instead, cases ought to be a good blend of experience and precept. Yet Kopelman does not deny the validity of some axioms arising from case experience. She quotes Hare on this point as follows:

6g

Descriptive premise:	The morally important points vary from case to case in medicine.
Inferential premise:	Weights about values and their importance vary from case to case.
Inductive Generalization:	Cases must be resolved on the basis of their own unique factors and parameters.

Learning from experience is not just empirical observation; it is the adoption of precepts or principles as a result of our reflection on what has happened to us.[20]

Hare's point is well-taken. Presumably this is Siegler's conviction as well, although it sometimes appears that each case is so unique, in his view, that no axioms could be extrapolated to the next case. At any rate Kopelman notes that the case-studies fallacies derive from several sources.

First, as methods of reasoning the concrete cases are so seductive that they may sway abstract convictions (which, we would add, is precisely their point). A good example of such swaying has been provided by Joanne Lynn, a physician who served on the staff of the president's commission. Her example is that, no matter how rational and thoroughly planned it may be, she can torpedo any national health-care policy by putting a little old lady who is not getting enough health care on television for five minutes!

The point to be pressed is that individual cases can appeal to emotions rather than to reason. In this sense, Daniel Callahan was incorrect when he argued in his Shattuck lecture that individual case analysis was easy compared to the formulation of public-policy medical ethics positions.[21] The fact is that resolving individual cases is far more difficult than formulating abstract policies, since the latter play with principles while the former play with individual lives.

Finally Kopelman notes that the case-studies, inductive approach can easily be misunderstood. One individual analyzed by a medical ethicist and physicians might become in their minds a paradigm of competency when others, who may be equally or surpassingly competent, "may not be as articulate."[22]

A number of thinkers view the inductive process as more than enriching the experience of the concrete. Rather it is needed to develop axioms and principles, as the quote from Hare, and the examples from Hooker and Cabot attest. Examples of inductive models of moral reasoning can be found in Thomasma,[23] Brody,[24] and McCullough,[25] among many others.

C. Guidelines for Reasoning

(1) Take McCullough's view as a case in point. Beginning with the question "How does one resolve conflicts among goods?" McCullough parallels the process of diagnostic reasoning by determining the balance of two perspectives on the patients' best interests, that of medicine and that of the patient.   In working through the case one is to be guided by the dictum that "No argument is to be taken as forever final, flawless and utterly convincing. Each is open to honest criticism and disagreement"[26]   (Again, we would note, just as diagnostic reasoning is.) McCullough emerges from the inductive process with a policy guiding decision-making by and for patients. His argument runs as shown in 6h.

6h	
Descriptive premise:	Cases must be resolved on an individual basis.
Inferential premise:	Although each case is different, some axioms derived from the case apply externally.
Inferential premise:	Since all of these have the potential to conflict with one another, no ultimate, forever true resolution can be made.
Inductive generalization:	Only a "strategy for conflict resolution" can be mapped out from a body of cases.
Axioms or policy:	(See below.)

McCullough's strategy for the resolution of conflict[27] is actually an inductive product that may later guide other case resolutions. It is a form of a scheme for weighting values, but does not require either rigid adherence or an oath of ultimate fealty. (We presume that Siegler would agree with it also.)

Nonetheless, from his other writings[28] one can assume that McCullough takes autonomy seriously. First, if the patient appeals to a strong preference or central value, then autonomy should guide the physician. If the patient has a reversible state of reduced autonomy, then the physician acts to reverse that state and then acts to implement patient preferences or values. If there is an irreversible reduction of autonomy, then the physician acts on the basis of the patients' value history. If that history cannot be obtained, then "the beneficence model should be determinative."[29]

In this example, autonomy predominates. Indeed, it may be the case that the "autonomy backdrop" present in this example is the clearest form of the backdrop providing the normative force to the conclusion. And yet there are some puzzling aspects to this example that do not permit us to draw such a straightforward conclusion.

First, the process does not lead inexorably to the primacy of the principle of autonomy, but rather, to the primacy of resolving issues on a case-by-case basis. Second, unlike Siegler's negotiated-values model, the process should be guided by experiential axioms in which good outcomes for the patient predominate (this seems to be an unexpressed premise of McCullough's argument, as is the next point). Good outcomes predominate when patient autonomy is respected. Hence, third, conflict resolution is best approached by promoting autonomy and patient values as far as possible.

(2) Another example can be drawn from the philosophical work of Pellegrino and Thomasma.[30] After arguing that the doctor-patient relation is the basis of a philosophy of medicine and its most crucial characteristic, they propose that the relationship is such that its purpose is healing. If healing is to take place, certain axioms must guide that healing. These axioms are regarded as ethical. Further they are thought to be derived from the nature of medicine itself, rather than being externally applied.[31] The axioms are: (1) Do no harm; (2) Respect the vulnerability of patients; (3) Treat each patient as a class instance of the human race. Their argument can be fleshed out as in 6i.

Pellegrino and Thomasma therefore argue that related axioms are embedded in medical practice as a result of the profession and commitment to heal and comfort. Their discussion makes it clear that the "Do no harm" axiom (or what is often called the principle of nonmaleficence) has come to have specific content in the thinking of professions -- it does not absolutely prohibit the inevitable harm which

<table>
<tr><td>6i</td><td></td></tr>
</table>

6i	
Descriptive premise:	The doctor-patient relation is the philosophical and ethical basis of medicine. Its object is healing.
Inferential premise:	Values come to play in the negotiation between doctor and patient.
Inductive generalization:	Yet not all the values are negotiable. Some are nonnegotiable (normative) if the healing aim of medicine is to take place.
Policy or set of axioms:	Nonnegotiable values are nonmaleficence, respect for patient vulnerability, and treating all patients equally. If any of these are violated, authentic healing does not occur.

accompanies surgical interventions (as long as the balance of good over evil likely to be accomplished is predominantly positive). However it does dictate against interventions about which the outcome is sufficiently uncertain and the primary motivation for acting is to "do something." Further, the weight given to this principle in traditional medical thinking serves to establish its priority when the general moral principle of nonmaleficence comes into conflict with other principles (such as the obligation to promote benefit for society or other individuals in the situation). These elements are claimed to arise directly from the context of practice in a way that shows they are not simply applications of additional general ethical principles.

The debate about this argument is fairly well developed. For example, Thomasma and Pellegrino, in the article cited, argue that axioms flow from the purpose of medicine itself. Six commentators discuss this claim, and the two authors respond in the same journal in "Response to Our Commentators,"[32] "Medicine as Action Theory,"[33] and "An Axiology of Medicine."[34] At the heart of most objections is (a) concern that this view of axioms falls victim to the "naturalistic fallacy," and/or (b) a question about whether health can function as a moral value.[35]

It is also important to note the difference between Pellegrino and Thomasma's argument and Siegler's. Both are derived from the doctor-patient relation. Both stress negotiation. But Pellegrino and Thomasma note limits on negotiation. The axioms derived from medicine as an art of healing give normative force to medical practice. Put another way, the axioms proposed are conditional. *If* medicine is to heal, it cannot violate or harm patients, perpetuate patient vulnerabilities (such as their loss of autonomy), or treat them unequally.

Further 6i differs from McCullough's approach (6h) because it provides content to resolutions through its axioms, whereas

McCullough's conflict-resolution model is still somewhat relativistic and contentless (one does not have to respect autonomy, necessarily).

D. An Inductive Process

Another fine example of the inductive origination model in which practice determines middle-level principles or axioms, is drawn from Stephen Toulmin's account of an ethics of discretion.[36] Toulmin argues that in a gross, impersonal age, ethics is in danger of becoming too generalized, too bureaucraticized, too remote from individual and family concerns. In particular he reacts as Tolstoy did, to the giant system of public-policy ethics, an ethics of strangers. In its place, Toulmin proposes that we substitute an "ethics of discretion." Discretionary ethics would be characterized by considerable leeway for making decisions (decisions made by those as close to the case as possible) and love.

Toulmin's article appeared before a number of other proposals that fit into his scheme. One, for example, was a proposal made by the Law Reform Commission of Canada that in making ethical decisions about dying patients, the conclusions and treatment plans developed by the patients with their families and doctors would be immune to subsequent prosecution.[37] This proposal was subsequently endorsed by the editor-in-chief[38] and some section editors[39] of the *Journal of the American Geriatrics Society*.

Another concrete example of an ethics of discretion along the lines of Toulmin's argument was Dr. Gene H. Stollerman's reaction to the Claire Conroy case discussed earlier. Reacting against the New Jersey Supreme Court ruling that decisions made about withholding food and water from dying nursing-home residents required consultation with two other physicians and the permission of the state's ombudsman office, Stollerman proposed that physicians must be free to do the "loving thing" in each situation.[40] Later Joseph Fletcher extrapolated this situational concept to the problem of assisting an early death for patients who request it.[41]

Filled in with these subsequent ideas, Toulmin's inductive approach might look like 6j.

At the start of the chapter, we noted that origination reasoning from practice to axioms was case driven, eclectic, analytically diverse, and axiomatic. Later we saw that some forms of argument posed only negotiation about values as axiomatic (the pure inductive examples by Siegler and the insight of psychology of medicine about the impact of disease on persons). A second form developed guidelines or a schema of preferred values in resolving conflicts (the McCullough example). Still others posit a series of non-negotiable, yet conditional axioms, that were formed from the process. The fourth type was found in our most recent example: an inductive process that led to an axiom about

6j

Descriptive premise:	Impersonal ethics do not do justice to the nuances of individual cases, and the myriad value components at stake in such cases.
Inferential premise:	Impersonal ethics must be supplanted by decision-making closer to the sources and consequences of the quandaries.
Inferential premise:	Discretionary space must be provided to responsible parties to bring about careful, even loving decisions.
Inductive generalization:	An ethics of discretion should replace an impersonal, bureaucratic ethics in health care.
Axioms or Policy:	The law should protect discretionary decisions made by doctors, patients, and families from subsequent investigation and litigation.

the correct type of ethics to be used in resolving problems in health care.

E. New Primary Principles

One step farther along the path of inductive models is the view that practice gives rise to new primary moral principles. Of course, there can be some question, about whether it is practice itself which gives rise to theory, or whether it is actually theory *about* practice or theory-laden practice which functions thus.

(1) Alasdair MacIntyre, in his article "Why Is the Search for the Foundations of Ethics So Frustrating?"[42] caps two previous articles on the problem of lack of moral consensus in our culture[43] by intimating that a social consensus creates new moral principles, although he qualifies this in *After Virtue*.[44] MacIntyre's argument comes at the social consensus question negatively. He tries to show that a lack of culturally accepted moral principles (the problem of pluralism) leads to moral dissolution in practice. (This seems to be in part why Engelhardt insists so much on autonomy -- so that one could not read "dissolution" but rather "improvement" in current conduct.) Modern citizens cannot agree about moral policies or action plans because they cannot agree in principle. This argument rests on several presuppositions which MacIntyre may also be trying to invalidate by his argument.

The first is that ethical reasoning must be proved deductively. If there can be no agreement on the starting principle, then, of course, there can be no agreement on conclusions (we have shown that this is not necessarily true). Second is the presupposition that pluralism necessarily leads to relativism. But it is not necessarily true that respect for a plurality of points of view means that all have equal, finite merit. Some positions are more nearly valid than others, especially if guidelines from a community of practice tilt some values over others (as MacIntyre himself suggests in *After Virtue*).

The third presupposition, however, is that social consensus about the primacy of certain values leads to the creation of new moral theories. Such a process would indeed exemplify origination reasoning giving rise to new primary moral principles. Let us look at one example of this occurrence in more detail.

Hardin's "lifeboat ethics" is a good case in point.[45] The current crisis of allocation of health care, Hardin argues, will require many changes in practice. These changes will be based on a whole complex set of values. After considerable experimentation, however, the crisis of allocation will lead to a new theory of moral choice. This theory will abandon fairness or equal treatment of individuals in favor of a new principle of survival of the fittest, however the latter may be interpreted -- that is, the fittest as the younger members of society, those with more to contribute (merit), or those with the best ability to pay. Thus, the appellation "lifeboat" ethics -- the weakest are hurled overboard.

(2) Another example of origination reasoning leading to the development of new moral theories is provided by the brilliant analysis made by Walter Burghardt in his introduction to Pedro Lain-Entralgo's *Therapy of the Word*.[46] There Burghardt traces the changes from a verbal to a pictorial culture occasioned by the rise of television. These changes are almost exactly the opposite from those that occurred as a mediaeval, pictorial culture met and often resisted the invention of the printing press. (One needs only note the way Reformers whitewashed the centuries-old, almost gaudily colorful paintings that covered the walls of their churches and cathedrals in favor of reading their Bibles.) The modern alteration back to a pictorial culture leads, among other things, to changes in the relationship between physician and patient. These changes, in turn, alter the fiduciary bond governing that relationship. Thus, as a consequence of social changes, Burghardt argues, a new principle of entrustment must now emerge.

(3) Indeed, the line of argument leading from social changes to a new social consensus to new moral theories and principles is commonly found in many thinkers. Recall Daniel Callahan's argument in his *The Tyranny of Survival*[47] that technological society creates the need for new moral principles. G. E. M. Anscombe, in her essay "Modern Moral Philosophy,"[48] details the change in the fundamental concepts of ethics from Aristotelian virtue theory to law theory as a result of cultural changes in the early centuries of the common era. Remember, too, Edmund Husserl's exploration of changes in the life-

world (the world of daily practice) that originated the very possibility of new ideas, even in disciplines as abstract as geometry.   For example, he argued that technological changes in perfecting the wheel were required before one could hypothesize a perfect circle.[49]

(4) Closer in some ways to medical patterns of reasoning in this approach are arguments, like those of sociobiologists, that new moral principles can be extracted from biological structures.   Most objectionable is the determinism of this point of view; less, perhaps, is the inductive process. Why so?

(5) The inductive process itself can furnish new insights about the philosophy of medicine. These insights, in turn, can be fashioned into an ethical theory governing medical transactions.   In their *A Philosophical Basis*, Pellegrino and Thomasma examine what they call the ontology of the body. In this ontology is a discussion of various activity levels of the body (social, personal, subconscious, etc.) and what happens to these levels, and to the person engaged in his or her body in interacting with the world, when disease strikes. From this descriptive analysis is drawn a concern for the vulnerability of the body, and consequently the person.   This "concern" can then be developed into an axiom and help feed into a general theory of clinical ethics whose emphasis is on addressing levels of vulnerability and need. A new moral theory of need and dependency, of justice and righting an imbalance is possible.

If this branch of origination reasoning is to offer a distinct alternative to the patterns of normative reasoning already discussed, it must be recognized that the "new" moral principles arise from the context of practice directly, rather than through the application of principles (as the major premise of a practical syllogism) to a new factual context. This latter activity might, indeed, yield a new minor premise, novel middle-level principles (what we call axioms), or dictates for action in the particular situation.

Earlier in this chapter we contrasted the tendency of followers of deductive models to weight and balance duties, rights, and values. In that process they often emerge with abstractions that fail to do justice to real human concerns.

F. Strengths of the Origination Model

A major strength of the origination model, therefore, is its reliance on the real-world, lived realities of medicine, especially as these are revealed in cases or in the negotiations that occur in the doctor-patient relation. As we parenthetically noted when discussing Loretta Kopelman's cautions about the case-studies approach, although the emotional content of individual cases may shape our generalizations, that is precisely the purpose of starting from the concrete and moving to the general. If one takes a more Aristotelian view, induction can lead to valid axioms and principles, as the quote from Hare attests and Pellegrino and Thomasma's conditional-axiom proposal works out.

If one takes a less sunny view of the process, one nevertheless arrives at a cautious set of claims derived from reality and experience, open to further revisions. These claims are not seen as quite so universally valid as Pellegrino and Thomasma's axioms. In logical terms, they are collective universals, statements that only cover the specific individuals studied. This seems to be what McCullough was driving at when he claimed that no solution would be final, and all would be subject to further revision. (We will examine this point again in our unitary theory in chapter 8.) Other thinkers fall on the cusp between inductive universal axioms and collective universal axioms. An example was run in Dr. Cabot's supposition that, although his data on truth telling was limited to his own eight-year study, that data was extrapolatable and could be verified by others.

A second major strong point of the origination model is its attempt to validate the ends or goals of the human enterprise of medicine as ethical. Recall that almost all the models involved in this chapter originate in cases, in interactions between doctors and patients. This interaction is assumed to be the primary focus of ethical import, the place where the needle hits the vinyl, so to speak. If this validation of medicine as a moral enterprise has any merit, then the moral weight of the inductive products can be derived from the realities of practice itself. We will examine the relation of medical ethics and medicine in our final chapter. For now it suffices to briefly analyze how it is possible that the inductive process can contain normative force. This is a third strength, if such an argument can be convincing.

The third strength of the origination model is therefore that it develops axioms from the goal of the medical discipline itself rather than from "external" axiomatic interpolation. Recall that a major weakness of deductive application and mediation models was that, in adhering perforce to a single theory or principle from which conclusions were to be derived, additional help seemed to be needed from "outside" the theory, help in the form of rules or other guidelines for action. Thus we were left either with the normative force of the principle without justifications for application or with justifications for applications but a concomitant destruction of the exclusivity of the single principle. No such problems occur in the origination model. The conclusion is reached using a collage of different, diverse axioms, themselves derived from the richness of reality. Further, extrapolation can leave behind the dangers of capriciousness and delineation noted by Kopelman. Thus, the normative force of the inductive product is not dependent on the context alone, as in the determination model.

Consequently this model can form the basis of revisions in professional ethics. It is no surprise then that many thinkers employing the inductive model have written on the topic of professional ethics.

But precisely how does the normative force come about in an inductive procedure? Let us look more carefully at the assumptions not clearly articulated in the inductive reasoning examples put forward in this chapter.

The best way to see what additional components be present in the ethical inductive process is to contrast it with a behavioral research study. Take a study of interactions by oncologists on rounds as an example.[50] Against the backdrop of a general theory of the importance of the doctor-patient relation, studies have been conducted that have proven that patients cannot evaluate the competency of their physician. As a consequence they tend to judge the quality of their doctor by "bedside manner," and other interpersonal skills. Apparently the "best" manner was found to be a serious, even negative voice tone coupled with a positive affect. In other words, physicians are judged good doctors by their seriousness and concern. They are judged by how they behave, not what they know.

Against this backdrop, then, an hypothesis is formed that behavior cannot be predicted on the basis of physician attitudes, and that it must be measured directly. Criteria and methods are established (observer reliability checks, patient sample, measurement scales, etc.), and direct observation of important behaviors is conducted. Among the behaviors are: discusses test results with patient, describes future treatment plans, engages in small talk, introduces self to patient, and provides verbal support. The inductive product from this study is that there is virtually no correlation between physicians' attitudes about cancer patients and their behaviors, or, even no correlation between their subjective judgments about which needs of the patient they addressed and what needs were actually addressed. One policy product would therefore be "that behavior cannot be inferred from paper and pencil measures and thus must be measured directly in the setting in which it occurs."[51] An axiom resulting from the study would be: greater emphasis on nonverbal communication skills is needed in health care.

Of course none of the conclusions carries normative force unless one considers possible harms to the patient that might come from lack of attention to his or her need. This is an important point because it brings us to the consideration of the roles of the "backdrop" as we have called it in deriving the normative force of the inductive process.

In those examples that are contentless the question of normative force is mute. The process yields only guidelines for open discussion, for fully negotiated and contracted values (Siegler) or even for an hierarchy of values that might be used (but not necessarily so) in

resolving conflicts (McCullough). For those examples that do yield
normative statements (Pellegrino and Thomasma, Toulmin), an
assumption is made that the descriptive premise carries in it some
hidden normative qualities.   At this point the ethical inductive
examples diverge from the descriptive study of oncology interactions,
for we do not consider the latter's descriptive premise about attitudes
and behavior to be anything more than that. Yet, as Thomasma and
Pellegrino argue, for example, the aim of the doctor-patient relation,
healing, is itself a moral enterprise.   The normative force of the
conditional axioms comes from that ethical perspective. Hence, we
would agree with Hare's perception that axioms and principles can be
partially derived from our experience, if the "experience" of which we
speak is properly delimited as carrying within it ethical values at
stake. Another way of putting this is that not all experiences from
which we derive inductive generalizations are inherently ethical, as our
oncology interaction example demonstrates.

More important for the normative force question, however, is the
role the backdrop plays in all our inductive examples. A hidden
assumption of both Hooker's and Cabot's arguments was that one
must not harm patients, the Hippocratic "primum non nocere," just as
we saw McCullough's not so hidden assumption was the importance
of autonomy (for the same reason). In the Pellegrino and Thomasma
argument, an assumption, spelled out elsewhere in their book, is that
one must act to assist human need. A professional must act to
reverse impairment. Further a health professional must make right
and good decisions with and for patients.[52]

We may conclude from these reflections that only a select few of
the inductive reasoning examples offer explicit reflection on the way
the inductive generalization possesses normative force.   These
examples are limited to processes in which the descriptive premise has
been circumscribed and its ethical components properly described.
According to "backdrop," however, all origination-model examples
derive a normative character for their inductive products from hidden
assumptions. In this respect, even the purely descriptive oncology
project has some normative quality if meeting patient needs and not
harming them is seen as the study's backdrop value system.

The fourth strength of the origination model is responsiveness to
cultural change in a way that the application model -- with its
assumption that moral principles are abstract and changeless -- for
example, is not. By contrast, MacIntyre's reflections on the problem
of agreements in a pluralistic age is quite acutely aware of the
fundamental impact of social change -- including alterations in the
possibilities for even establishing fundamental moral principles. As we
saw, analyses of aspects of society by Callahan, Hardin, Anscombe,
Husserl, and others must be incorporated into any general bioethical

theory.

The fifth strength of origination reasoning is that it need not (and usually does not) respond to cultural change by degenerating into an anarchical form of ethical relativism. It attempts to retain the principled character of the moral life by considering what fundamental principles are newly indicated by the new dimensions of social life now budding forth.

A final strength is that the same methods that are employed by inductive scholars to derive new moral theories or axioms, can also be employed to derive cross-cultural moral theories. In the ideal, then, the new principles to be drawn from practice will include both a response to social change and a response to existing cultural diversity.

The chief question that can be raised about the branch of the origination model that rests on social analysis as its base is whether it is really (as it purports to be) merely a description of social practice or whether, instead, it is based on a theory about social practice, as is for example, a quantitative measurement theory (like our oncology study example), or Marxist analysis.[53] If such an approach does, indeed, rest on a theory about practice then it is likely that a fundamental aspect of the theory with which it is laden is itself normative. If this is the case, then there is no clear alternative to the application model in this pattern of reasoning.

If this is not the case, then the naturalistic fallacy charges arise against origination with a vengeance.

G. Weaknesses of the Origination Model

Despite the efforts we have made to detail ways the normative force might come from the descriptive premise, objections to the origination model center around the naturalistic fallacy or the contentlessness of the process. We will examine four such weaknesses: (1) that the *ought* is derived from what *is*; (2) if that is not the case, then the descriptive premise must assume that healing, meeting human needs, or reversing impairments are all ethical values from which the normative content of the process can be derived; (3) that this model neglects links with ethical theory and abstract truths; (4) and finally, that the model, if contentless, leads to bureaucratic, procedural ethics.

Objection 1: Like the other inductive model we have already examined, this one seems to fall victim to the naturalistic fallacy objection. This objection applies if one claims that the normative force of the conclusions reached stems from the descriptive premises.

Objection 2: We noted how some thinkers derive that normative force from ambient considerations rather than trying to argue that the ethical nature of the conclusions flow from the premises. If that tack is taken, however, the inductive model cannot remain inductive *per se*.

Instead, origination reasoning would be a sort of modified inductive account in which the premises contributed to, but did not "induce," the conclusion. Among the ambient considerations would be ethical principles "floating about" in one's culture, or more explicit norms serving as backdrop to the discussion. An example of the former would be a discussion of the correct model of the doctor-patient relation, let us say the dialogical model, in which a description of what works best leads to the conclusions. Yet the hidden prescript floating about in this analysis might be the principle of autonomy's requirement that persons be free to determine their own course of treatment. An example of the second way in which norms influence inductive reasoning would be the same discussion about the proper nature of the doctor-patient relation. Instead of ignoring the backdrop principles, this approach might recognize the importance of nonmaleficence in the manner used by Pellegrino and Thomasma.

Yet, ethical skeptics (like Kai Nielsen), ethical relativists, and situation ethicists would criticize even this minimalist normative approach as making too much of ethical principles. Why mediate one's response to a medical situation by means of abstract social analysis and concern for implicit or explicit backdrop precepts? Instead why not respond directly to the morally relevant features of the specific situation?

The answer to this objection might be that those "morally relevant features" themselves do, in fact, function as the source for the normative force of the inductive process. Thus the healing aim of medicine, caring for the patients' vulnerability, or meeting human needs, are normative precepts hidden in the morally relevant features of cases. Further, these features are sufficient to provide the normative elements of the inductive products derived from the descriptive premises. This response, however, requires more work than has been accomplished to date on the ethical nature of the healing aims of medicine.

Objection 3:   The third objection comes at the origination approach from the other side. This objection states that this model neglects the power of general ethical theory and abstract truths. Earlier we asked why we should choose the realities of the context rather than important ethical theories. Would not the former be less important than the latter? Part of the answer to this challenge lies in the idealist or realist proclivities of individuals. But another part of the answer stems from the practical nature of medicine (and perforce, clinical ethics). Each case is like a moving picture. Prominent values one day may lose their prominence the next with some new onslaught to the patient. As a consequence, major attention must be paid to clinical realities and the ever-changing health professional-patient relation, as well as to its institutional context.

Paying attention to practice does not necessarily mean abandoning concern for general ethical truths. As has been underlined already, the origination model almost always leads to new theory or new axioms. It does not accept their *a priori* validity without prior descriptive analysis.

Objection 4: In an age of pluralism, there is a great danger of neglecting content in favor of formalism. The inductive approach falls victim to this objection more than deductive models, since it starts with a sort of contentlessness (unless, of course, it acknowledges normative contents in its premises, but then it is not purely inductive). Nonetheless, Colleen Clements has pointed out that Engelhardt, Veatch, and even Beauchamp and Childress are subject to the same critique[54] (even though they are hardly inductive ethicists).

For Engelhardt, bioethics must focus on procedures for protecting the autonomy of individuals in a pluralistic society, even though the good or bad consequences of their autonomous actions are left open. [55] In order to avoid "imposing" strictures on anyone, Engelhardt holds that a "bureaucratic and procedural character of modern bioethics" would be nonpartisan with respect to moral viewpoints.[56] Veatch's procedural ethics is the contract or covenant between doctor and patient, the nature of which is left open, although justice functions as its backdrop.[57] Beauchamp and Childress offer formal conditions for action guides, such as universalizability, that they describe as necessary conditions for moral thinking. These, too, are contentless.[58]

The danger of a formalist, procedural, bureaucratic public-policy ethic is that it inordinately focuses on human freedom, patient autonomy, and informed consent as preconditions for ethics rather than as values, among others, to be negotiated in the context. This is detrimental to medicine which must pay most attention to acting in the best interests of patients.[59] Further, the bureaucratic ethics that results becomes too far removed from the drama and values of individuals. It becomes an ethic of rules that, ironically, circumscribe the very freedom needed to make moral judgments.

As we pointed out earlier in this chapter, origination reasoning need not succumb to relativism and formalism. In fact, its response to pluralism is ethically sounder than deductive ethics. The latter seemingly has only two responses -- imposition of a principle not held by others to reach a conclusion, or retreat into contentlessness to preserve a fundamental moral principle (such as autonomy) by making it a condition of possibility for ethics rather than part of the normative enterprise. The origination model, on the other hand, is more sensitive to plurality just by reason of its inductive premises. These have been inaugurated in practice and their products return to practice. Thus their "content" remains ethically relevant to components of life and the practice of medicine.

H. Conclusion

The origination model points to another missing component in deductive reasoning models -- the individual's virtue. If experience with the realities of clinical medicine in its social context require sophisticated respect for the individual and social values of one's time and place, and the power of discerning right from wrong in developing new moral theories or axioms, then individual virtue must also be placed in a general theory of medical ethics. Of all models it is the least talked-about by ethicists, but the most-stressed in the clinical setting, professional schools, professional codes, and in our public and private training grounds for citizenship, our schools and churches. The virtue model is examined next.

NOTES

1. H. Worthington Hooker, *Physician and Patient* (New York: Baker and Scribner, 1849), p. 362.

2. Ibid., p. 370.

3. Ibid., p. 370.

4. Ibid., p. 372.

5. Ibid., p. 359.

6. Ibid., p. 368.

7. Ibid., p. 380.

8. "Thoughts from the Heart," *Stethoscope*, the newspaper of Loyola University of Chicago Medical Center. (May 1986), 2.

9. Sissela Bok, *Lying: Moral Choice in Public and Private Life* (New York: Vintage Books, 1979), pp. 215-230.

10. Beauchamp and Childress, *Principles of Biomedical Ethics*.

11. Richard C. Cabot, "The Use of Truth and Falsehood in Medicine: An Experimental Study," *American Medicine* 5 (1903), 344-349.

12. Ibid., 349.

13. Ibid.

14. Eric Cassell, "The Relief of Suffering," *Archives of Internal Medicine* 143, no. 3 (March 1983), 522-523; Eric Cassell, "The Nature of Suffering and the Goals of Medicine, *New England Journal of Medicine* 306, no. 11 (18 March 1982), 639-645; cf. Bergsma with Thomasma, *Health Care: Its Psychosocial Dimensions*.

15. Mark Siegler, "Searching for Moral Certainty in Medicine," *Bulletin of the New York Acadademy of Medicine* 57 (1981), 57-69.

16. Pellegrino and Thomasma, *For the Patients' Good*, chapter 4.

17. Siegler, "Searching for Moral Certainty in Medicine," pp. 61-62.

18. Howard Brody, *Ethical Decisions in Medicine* 2nd edition (Boston: Little, Brown, and Co., 1981), p. 35.

19. Loretta Kopelman, "Teaching Commentary: The Case Method and the Case-Method Fallacy," *Society for Health and Human Values Notes* (Now *Bulletin*) 15 (February 1985), 2-3.

20. R. M. Hare, "Principles," *Proceedings of the Aristotelian Society* 73 (1972-73), 1-18.

21. Daniel Callahan, "Shattuck Lecture -- Contemporary Biomedical Ethics," *New England Journal of Medicine* 302, no. 22 (May 29, 1980), 1228-1233.

22. Kopelman, "Teaching Commentary," 3.

23. David C. Thomasma, "Training in Medical Ethics: An Ethical Workup," *Forum on Medicine* 1, no. 9 (December 1978), 30-33.

24. Howard Brody, *Ethical Decisions in Medicine*.

25. Laurence B. McCullough, "Addressing Ethical Dilemmas: An Ethics Workshop," *The New Physician* 33 (October 1984), 34-35.

26. Ibid., 34.

27. Ibid.

28. See, for example, Laurence B. McCullough and Stephen Wear,

"Respect for Autonomy and Medical Paternalism Reconsidered," *Theoretical Medicine* 6, no. 3 (October 1985), 295-308.

29. McCullough, "Addressing Ethical Dilemmas," 34.

30. Pellegrino and Thomasma, *A Philosophical Basis of Medical Practice*, chapter 8.

31. Edmund D. Pellegrino and David C. Thomasma: "Philosophy of Medicine as the Source for Medical Ethics."

32. Edmund D. Pellegrino and David C. Thomasma: "Response to Our Commentators."

33. Edmund D. Pellegrino and David C. Thomasma: "Medicine as a Science of Action," *Metamedicine* 2 (1981), 235-243.

34. Edmund D. Pellegrino and David C. Thomasma: "Toward an Axiology for Medicine," *Metamedicine* 2 (1981), 235-243.

35. Dutch critics and the response of Thomasma and Pellegrino to them can be found in David C. Thomasma and Edmund D. Pellegrino, "Challenges for a Philosophy of Medicine of the Future: A Response to Fellow Philosophers in the Netherlands," *Theoretical Medicine* 8, no. 2 (June 1987), 187-204 (edited by Henk ten Have, Jurrit Bergsma and Jan Broekman). Additional critiques were provided by Dutch scholars in the Dutch journal of medicine, with a subsequent response: David C. Thomasma and Edmund D. Pellegrino, "De filosofische basis van de geneeskunde," *Nederlands Tijdschrift voor Geneeskunde* 130 (1986), 1495-1497.

36. Stephen Toulmin, "The Tyranny of Principles."

37. Law Reform Commission of Canada, *Euthanasia, Aiding Suicide and Cessation of Treatment*. Report 20 (Ottawa: Minister of Supply and Services of Canada, 1983).

38. Gene H. Stollerman, "Editorial: Lovable Decisions, Rehumanizing Dying," *Journal of the American Geriatrics Society* 34 (February 1986), 172-174.

39. Gene H. Stollerman, "Editorial: Quality of Life: Treatment Decisions and the Third Alternative," *Journal of the American Geriatrics Society* 32 (July 1984), 483-484; John R. Ball, "Withholding Treatment: A Legal Perspective," *Journal of the American Geriatrics Society* 33 (July 1984), 528-531; David C. Thomasma, "Ethical Judgments of Quality of Life in the Care of the Aged," *Journal of the American Geriatrics Society* 33 (July 1984), 525-527. For responses, see John Sorenson, "The Character of Life to Guide Rehumanizing Dying," *Journal of the American Geriatrics Society* 35 (March 1987), 262-263; Joanne Lynn, "Comment on Lovable Decisions," *Journal of the American Geriatrics Society* 35 (March 1987), 272.

40. Gene H. Stollerman, "The Right to Serve and the Limits of Autonomy," *Journal of the American Geriatrics Society* 35 (July 1987), 702; David C. Thomasma, "Caveat Philosophus: Technology's Abuse-Potential in the Decision to Terminate Life," *Journal of the American Geriatrics Society* 35 (July 1987), 703-704.

41. Joseph Fletcher, "Medical Resistance to the Right to Die," *Journal of the American Geriatrics Society* 35 (July 1987), 679-682.

42. Alasdair MacIntyre, "Why Is the Search for the Foundations of Ethics So Frustrating?" *Hastings Center Report* 9 (1979), 16-22.

43. Alasdair MacIntyre, "How Virtues Become Vices: Values, Medicine and Social Context"; Alasdair MacIntyre, "Patients as Agents."

44.   Alasdair MacIntyre, *After Virtue* (Notre Dame: Notre Dame University Press, 1981).

45.   Garret Hardin, "Lifeboat Ethics: The Case Against Helping the Poor," *Psychology Today* 8 (1974), 38-43; and "Living on a Lifeboat, " *Bioscience* 24 (October 1974), 561-568.

46.   Pedro Lain Entralgo, *Therapy of the Word in Classical Antiquity*, ed. and trans. L. J. Rather and John M. Sharp (New Haven: Yale University Press, 1970).

47.   Daniel Callahan, *The Tyranny of Survival and Other Pathologies of Civilized Life* (Lanham, MD: University Press of America, 1985).

48.   G. E. M. Anscombe, "Modern Moral Philosophy," *Philosophy* 33 (1958), 1-19.

49.   Edmund Husserl, *Phenomenology and the Foundations of the Sciences*, trans. Ted Klein and William Pohl (The Hague/Hingham, MA: Martinus Nijhoff, 1980).

50.   C. Blanchard, J. Ruckdeschel, E. Blanchard, J. Arena, N. Saunders, and E. Drew Malloy, "Interactions Between Oncologists and Patients During Rounds," *Annals of Internal Medicine* 99 (1983), 694-699.

51.   *Ibid.*, 699.

52.   Pellegrino and Thomasma, *A Philosophical Basis of Medical Practice*, chapter 7.

53.   Annemick Richters and Eduard Bonsel, "The Judgment Comes with Healing in its Wings: A Call for Rational Detachment," *Theoretical Medicine* 8, no. 2 (June 1987), 147-162.

54.   Colleen Clements, "The Bureau of Bioethics: Norm Without Content Is Meaningless," *Perspectives in Biology and Medicine* 27 (Winter 1984), 171-182.

55.   H. Tristram Engelhardt, Jr., "Bioethics in Pluralist Societies," *Perspectives in Biology and Medicine* 26 (1982), 64-78.

56.   Ibid., 70.

57.   R. Veatch, *A Theory of Medical Ethics*, pp. 324-330.

58.   Beauchamp and Childress, *Principles of Biomedical Ethics*.

59.   Pellegrino and Thomasma, *For the Patient's Good*.

CHAPTER SEVEN
The Virtue Model[*]

Thus far, we have concentrated on the "what" of moral action -- on ways to determine *what to do* in situations of choice. This focus is typical of most contemporary discussions in ethical theory and medical ethics. The case is presented, and the question on everyone's mind is "what is the proper thing to do?" The debate we have dealt with in previous chapters relates to the most adequate way of answering this question -- whether by application of principles "from above," or by induction "from below" responding to elements of the context of action and moving towards principles, or by some intermediate method.

However, there are other important elements in the moral life; and this exclusive focus on **what to do** tends to obscure them. Morality addresses, not only what actions we should perform (and those which we should refrain from performing), it also has to do with **the kind of person we should each strive to become.** This is the arena of the virtues. We are concerned, for example, not only with determining and doing "the honest thing" but with becoming and being "an honest person." Health professionals are not only concerned with acting rightly for patients, but also with the moral character of those who responsibly care for patients.

A. The Definition of Virtue
Two contemporary descriptions from the medical ethics literature deal with the idea of virtue. Both, however, concentrate too much on the motive of an act. Consider Gregory Pence's characterization of the concept: "the heart of ethics in daily life is having such a character that one wants to do the morally right act."[1] Thus, virtue has to do primarily with *motives*. Pence analyzes virtues in terms of three components, at least two of which primarily involve the affective dimension. As he summarizes his analysis:

> First, they [the virtues] are dispositions to act. Second, they are dispositions to feel that result from good character, which is a mean between extremes of character. Third, virtues are acquired by educating emotions through thought.[2]

---

[*] The authors are indebted to John David Grayson for his assistance in drafting this chapter.

A second example comes from of Jonsen and Hellegers for whom virtues are:

> rationally intended, effectively rooted attitudes whereby persons consistently seem to incline toward certain sorts of behavior. Terms such as benevolence, honesty, trustworthiness, and sobriety [describe] particular modes of these states of character.[3]

Thus, the virtues seem at first blush to describe *motivation* to do good deeds, rather than describe the good deeds themselves.

The precise role of the affective dimension here is far from clear. On one reading of Pence's initial characterization, for example, it would appear that the *only* morally worthy motive is a desire to do what is right for its own sake -- thus the one and only virtue would be *conscientiousness*.   But, as Frankena points out (following Prichard), it is questionable whether this is what we typically mean by *virtue* at all.[4]   Frankena and Prichard would call this "moral goodness" and distinguish it from "various other good motives or desires rooted in emotions like gratitude, benevolence, or courage."[5] In courage, for example, the passion involved is fear: the timid person feels excessive fear; the rash person feels a deficiency of fear; the courageous person feels the appropriate measure of fear.

This sort of example supports Pence's endorsement of Aristotle's "doctrine of the mean" -- the view that virtuous motives consist of an intermediate degree of feeling, avoiding extremes of excess and deficiency.   However, in general, this doctrine is fraught with difficulties.

As with most philosophical concepts, there is controversy about how to define a virtue (as well as about what traits count as virtues, the relation between various virtues, etc.).   Aquinas following Aristotle defined virtue as "a good operative habit."[6] The term "good" stood to distinguish virtue from vice, a bad operative habit. This points to the *normative* dimension of both general and specific virtue concepts. We call "virtues" only those traits which we find admirable. "Operative" stood for an increasing potential to act in a certain way (for Aristotle the virtues activated already existing tendencies of human psychology and made them stronger, thereby perfecting them).

Psychological potentialities in persons point to another conceptual requirement: that virtues be manifest in action. Although one's interior state of mind and heart is an important component of the virtues, it is not the only one. Virtues cannot typically be *wholly* interior affairs. Someone who claims that his "heart is in the right place" but who consistently fails to *act* accordingly when the occasion presents itself would not be credited as truly possessing the virtue in question. For example, one who *says* "I believe in forthrightly saying what is on my mind" but regularly shrinks from direct communication in difficult situations does not possess the trait of candor. She may *wish* she were a candid person. Perhaps she is even on the way to *becoming* a candid person. But the trait of candor is not yet operative within her. A "habit" was, in Aquinas's view, the perduring training of the passions, emotions, and the mind towardsthe good. Today we might call this the interiorization or individuation of externally molded training into character.

Three elements seem to be central to our concept of virtues, then: (a) that they are established or settled *dispositions* to act in certain ways, (b) that they are involved with the affective dimension of the person (although not exclusively), and (c) that they give rise to actions that are judged objectively good. Analysis of motives can color the quality of actions, but the actions themselves can and must be analyzed independent of motives as well. This point is very important for fitting the virtue theory into the other models thus far explored.

The key problem engaging us in this chapter is to determine the proper role of attention to character in medical ethics -- especially, where does it fit in relation to the intersection between theory and practice that we have been examining throughout this volume? Several possibilities exist.

B. Role of Virtues in Theory and Practice
1) Supplement or "add-on" (or "tack-on"): The most popular view is probably to see issues of character as external to the basic questions of theory. In this view the virtues function as a *supplement* to standards of right action. Pence's characterization could be read to suggest this view. First, we determine "the morally right act" (following one or a combination of the models discussed in previous chapters). At this point, the task of moral philosophers is probably completed; but medical educators or social-policy makers might go further to articulate structures which would motivate behavior to correspond to the guidelines that have been developed (i.e., arranging it so that "one wants to do" the action in question).

(a) *Reward or Punishment*: One instrument by which this is achieved is through a system of punishment. Here the "tacked-on" nature of this matter is obvious: to the weight of moral obligation is added a threat of social sanction for violating the standard of action or some other incentive to right action.

Within medical ethics, several areas of law are often appealed to in this way: (1) the criminal law may contain prohibitions against certain medical procedures, such as active euthanasia, and the punishment for doing this act is a matter for criminal prosecution.[7] Proposed measures to make abortion once again impermissible will also change the criminal code if enacted;   (2) professional licensure also includes prohibited actions. For example, Tennessee's "Right to Natural Death" statute declares that failure to honor a patient's Living Will may be punished by revocation of one's professional license; (3) malpractice actions, the threat of which is constantly in the mind of many practitioners today, tend to curtail some actions (e.g., paternalism) while encouraging others (e.g., repeated and sometimes unnecessary tests).

(b) *Economic Incentives*: Also in this same general realm are authors who focus on *economic incentives* to action which they regard as appropriate. For example, proponents of HMOs and DRGs often argue that cost-plus reimbursement and fee-for-service financing arrangements incorporate economic incentives to overtreat, whereas the structures they recommend incorporate countervailing incentives. Of course, these claims may be disputed. These same or related economic incentives are also seen by some as working against traditional medical and professional ethics. For example, the American Medical Association's Council on Ethical and Judicial Affairs has warned against HMO and PPO incentives in the form of bonuses to physicians to encourage them to avoid expensive tests and treatments. The reason is that the good of patients may suffer harm in such a scheme.[8]

(c) *Moral Education*: Another area in which attention to issues of motive and character might be relegated as a supplement to ethical reasoning is the domain of moral education -- either as part of childhood development or, perhaps, in the process of professional education. Nowadays, the most popular form of this approach is to call for "role models" among educators, where what they are expected to exemplify is not so much modes of ethical *reasoning* as seriousness of purpose in putting ethical rules and principles into *practice*. The presupposition of this approach is an *imitative* model of moral development.

These views of elements of virtue as "tacked-on" are unsatisfying, however. In the last analysis, they do not foster true *virtue* at all. Surely the settled disposition (a) to avoid social and legal sanctions is not a virtue. The settled disposition to obey the law from a motive of respect for the law in itself and the social system of laws is, indeed, a trait we would admire. But this (law-abidingness or respect for law) is quite different from acting from fear of sanctions -- a species of prudentialism which we might call C.Y.A. ("Cover Your Anatomy"). And the threat of legal sanctions does nothing to foster this admirable trait.   Similarly, a settled disposition (b) to respond to economic incentives is, at best, prudentialism (and perhaps cupidity). This is not a particularly admirable trait.   Nor is it clear that a settled disposition (c) among adults to imitate the patterns of action one has observed in role models is a trait that should be admired -- especially if it is a matter of blind imitation, unaccompanied by insight into the moral *point* of acting in this way.[9]   And yet it is this unreflective imitation that is all too often promoted in medical education. One of the authors once observed a teaching physician announce: "I don't care about what the textbooks say. I would never perform procedure *x* without confirmation of the diagnosis by test *y* -- and **I expect you to do likewise in your practice.**" No further rationale for this departure from standard practice was provided.

The ethics of precept and example, so often promoted in medical education, is actually not an ethics of freedom. It does not represent an interior disposition to do good in the sense of a fully formed moral person. For the idea of virtue, of "interior disposition," is correlated with the lack of external controls. Persons will act virtuously because they are so disposed, not because their role models tell them to act this way or because they wish to imitate their role models. The last point is also important. One may wish to imitate the life of a saint, say in courage and fortitude, but the role model is held up for one's own personal development. Such virtues will come from within the formed person, and not just by externally imitating the actions of the saint.   The same holds true of role model education.   The good physician is one who acts from interior motivation and disposition, even if the desire to act this way was once prompted (and/or is now supported) by the excellent standards set by the profession or role models.

Is it not possible for virtues to have a closer relationship to standards of action than from external copying? If we move away from an exclusive focus on the motivational element of virtues and pay more attention to their cognitive and objective aspects, other, more satisfactory forms of supplementation are possible. One thing that is meant by the injunction to honor "the spirit of the law" rather than merely "the letter" can be explicated by means of the role of settled traits of character. This is what Graber and his physician coauthors were getting at with regard to medical confidentiality, for example, when they said the following:

> Formal procedural safeguards might be devised to enforce some aspects of these rules of decorum, i.e., to prevent hospital employees other than those directly involved in the patient's care from having access to the chart. However, these could never be "fail safe," and they involve a greater loss (by impeding communication between those with a need to exchange information) than the gain to be achieved. *There is no substitute for morally sensitive behavior by the individuals involved.*[10]

Henry Beecher expresses a parallel sentiment with regard to human experimentation in the following passage:

> After some years of careful study of the available codes of the past which have been established to guide the medical investigator and after earnest attempts to write down a comprehensive code, the writer has had to conclude that it is not possible to lay down very many "rules" in terms of a code which can govern experimentation in man. In most cases these are more likely to do harm than good. Rules will not curb the unscrupulous.
>
> It is the writer's point of view that the best approach concerns the character, wisdom, experience, honesty, imaginativeness and sense of responsibility of the investigator who, in all cases of doubt or where serious consequences might remotely occur, will call in his peers and get the benefit of their counsel. Rigid rules will jeopardize the research establishments of this country where experimentation in man is essential.[11]

Ingelfinger's discussion of the virtues in health professionals makes a similar point. He argues that despite all standards and rules, federal guidelines and commands, if the particular health professional does not possess the virtues necessary to interiorize these objective rules and standards, then they will not be carried out.[12]

In both the cases cited, what is recommended is instilling tendencies (or strengthening those already present in inchoate form)--the interior disposition to *care* about certain things: the privacy of the patient, in the first case; the research subject's safety and welfare, in the second; patient welfare in Ingelfinger's position. The assumption is that reliance on discerning judgment guided by these concerns will be more reliable as a guide to action than any compendium of detailed policies that could be developed through the models of ethical reasoning discussed in earlier chapters. Thus the *principles* of confidentiality and protection of research subjects (which themselves would be established through one of the earlier reasoning modes) are supplemented in practice by internalized dispositions incorporating modes of both thought and feeling.

2) Mediation: Instead of just being tacked on, perhaps virtues might play a mediating role, much like that of mediation-model reasoning from theory to practice discussed in chapter 2 above. Thus when a conflict of principles arises, a virtuous person might resolve the conflict by an appeal to "the heart" rather than "the head." That is to say, he or she might respond to a situation as prompted by feelings stemming from settled traits of character rather than either appealing to intellectual intuition or trying to develop a rational priority principle. Note that this requires a view of virtues as involving more than a motivational "push" in a direction suggested by "external" reason. Instead, virtues must have cognitive content as well as emotional.

Indeed, the point of interiorization of external principles, axioms, and rules is to permit an individualized assessment of a situation, a process closely related to clinical hunches or gut feelings, a process far more complicated than a computerized decision-analysis tree. In effect, a virtuous person interprets a situation rapidly and coherently. He or she may not be able to provide reasons for the act that satisfy others ("The heart has its reasons . . . .") Nonetheless, the situational context has been interpreted in terms of possibilities for the good. Compare a virtuous person's response to an accident victim's plight with, say, that of a hardened thief. Where the virtuous person would first notice the victim's suffering and injuries, would react to these emotionally with empathy, and would respond to them by arranging aid, the thief would notice first the fat wallet lying by the individual, would respond to this with feelings of greed, and would react by snatching up the wallet and running away.

Thus, it is not simply a matter of an appeal to the heart, if what is meant by such an appeal is to emotive aspects of human character. The heart is not cognitive. Yet for the famous virtue theorists such as Aristotle and Saint Thomas Aquinas, the virtues infused, not just the emotions, but practical and theoretical reason itself. All human potentialities were capable of being habitualized towardsthe good. Thus, prudence, justice, fortitude, and temperance, the cardinal virtues, had to do with practical tendencies in human beings towardsthe good. In this system, as we saw prudence was in fact seen as the conclusion of a practical syllogism (the prudential act itself seen as the very definition of ethics). Wisdom, knowledge, and science were seen as intellectual virtues informing the mind and the will.[13] Thus, it would be a mistake to identify an interior disposition with a feeling. It is much more than that. Nonetheless, virtues are clearly accompanied by feelings.

For example, our physician who is a committed opponent of abortion might nevertheless find himself "tempted" to perform an abortion in a situation in which continuing the pregnancy threatens the life of the mother; and this temptation would be experienced by him, not as a purely intellectual insight or intuition, but rather as a focused urging of compassion. Here the principle of respect for life (and undoubtedly its corresponding virtue) is in conflict with itself in application to the different parties in the situation, and it is another settled trait of character which mediates the conflict. Often physicians speak of clinical hunches and gut feelings when discussing the vagaries of clinical judgment. There is a sense in which appeals to these intuitions helps to mediate difficult moral judgments between two good actions.

Vices can, of course, play the same role as virtues here: one who regularly felt himself drawn to the alternative which was most *profitable for himself* whenever faced with a choice between two or more treatment modalities that are equally justifiable on clinical grounds would be said to be *improperly* influenced by the vice of greed or cupidity.

The first code of ethics of the American Medical Association suggested that the personal virtue of the physician might, in general, play this sort of mediating role. Although admitting that "interpretation of these principles by an appropriate authority will be required at times" (presumably involving something like application-model reasoning), they go on to insist that:

> as a rule . . . the physician who is capable, honest, decent, courteous, vigilant, and an observer of the Golden Rule, and who conducts his affairs in the light of his own conscientious interpretation of these principles will find no difficulty in the discharge of his professional obligations.[14]

The term "interpretation" in this passage suggests the need for intellectual exercises of one or more of the sorts we have discussed earlier; but, since "conscientiousness" is perhaps itself a virtue (Frankena and Prichard notwithstanding) and is associated in this passage with a number of other obvious virtues, it is possible that what is meant here is more a matter of the "heart" than of the "head." If so, then this is an example of a virtues-as-mediation view. The discerning judgment employed in these interpretations is itself viewed as a component of the virtues in question. A similar view is expressed in Francis Peabody's hallowed article, "The Care of the Patient": "one of the essential qualities of the clinician is interest in humanity, for the secret of the care of the patient is in caring for the patient."[15]

3) Substitute: The strongest role that could be assigned to virtues is as an independent guide to action -- a substitute for principles, and rules. and for the modes of reasoning discussed in preceding chapters. Here the mode of decision-making would be as much affective as explicitly cognitive -- a matter of following the urgings of feelings or discerning judgments which are rooted in disciplined emotions or similar settled traits of character without any overt reasoning processes of the sort analyzed at length in earlier chapters.

It is important to distinguish the substitute role discussed below from an automatic role, the likes of which are detailed by John Graner. Graner holds that the modern physician's role has been reduced from that of action, the expression of oneself in a unique way to others, to labor. A laborer is one who is forced to function in a reproducible, interchangeable manner. This changeover in medicine occurred with the appearance of Descartes's ideas about the human body. At this time, the ascendancy of work (fabrication) over action occurred as an inevitable result of scientific achievements in understanding and technology.[16] Thus, the laborization of society has brought to the medical profession the "degrading element of replaceability."[17] If Graner's insight is correct, as we think it is, then it would be tempting to think that habitual action or disposition, that caused by the virtues, was a form of laborization rather than action as defined by Aristotle and as used by Graner. This is not the case. Rather, the virtues can be seen as substitutions for externally imposed standards. Let us look at this point more carefully.

Pence clearly holds a substitution version of a virtues approach in the following passage. He makes it clear that he not only believes that a virtues approach can serve as a substitute for an approach such as the "contract" model of the professional-patient relationship articulated most notably by Robert Veatch, but he is convinced that it is a *superior* approach.

> The best argument why contractualism is not the ideal, is that patients really want to be treated by physicians who practice the virtues. Contractualism falls short of the ideal for physician-patient relationships because people expect more of physicians as soon as problems arise. They expect virtues. Patients, if they could conceivably contract for these character traits, would want physicians who are competent, courageous, compassionate, honest, temperate, and so on. . . . Faced with choosing between a virtuous physician who does not enter into contracts and one who honors every detail of his contract but in everything else lacks compassion and honesty, few patients would opt for the contract.[18]

What is the difference between these two approaches? The advantages Pence and others see in a virtues approach appear to lie chiefly in two elements: comprehensiveness and spontaneity.

Comprehensiveness: A practitioner who has internalized the virtue of candor will not limit truth telling to those occasions and those items of information which are specified in some (written or unwritten) contract. Instead, she will *always* tell *the whole* truth in *all* her dealings with patients, families, and others. Lying, evasion, deception, calculated disclosure, and the like will be foreign to her nature. She will find forthrightness and openness the natural thing to do on every occasion.

This would be a refreshing contrast to discussions we hear repeatedly among practitioners nowadays about precisely what pieces of information must be revealed in order to satisfy the legal and contractual requirement of information disclosure. Furthermore, this requirement is often identified with the process of obtaining informed consent for surgery or other momentous procedures, and thus information sharing is often postponed until the occasion for obtaining a formal consent arises.

In contrast, the habitually candid physician would find it natural to share whatever information she possessed as she came into possession of it, not to wait for some formal occasion to make a carefully structured (and perhaps rehearsed) "disclosure."

Spontaneity: The other element that is particularly appealing about behavior stemming from a deep-seated and settled trait of character is its naturalness and spontaneity. There is something disconcerting about the thought that our physician deliberates and calculates about what information to share with us. We would prefer to think of him as an open person who communicates spontaneously, who finds it the natural thing to do to share with us what information he has about our condition.

Similarly, the thought of compassion being made a matter of the calculated and planned application of psychosocial techniques is disconcerting to patients. We would prefer to think of our physician's efforts in this direction as the spontaneous expression of feelings of compassion rather than an artifice or technique. Indeed, calculated compassion corresponds to one of the modes identified by MacIntyre "by which what have been virtues in one social and cultural context can become vices in another"[19]:

> the case where a disposition valuable for its own sake and valued for its own sake, as any genuine virtue must be (it may of course also be valued for further ends it serves) comes to be valued only or primarily for its employment as part of a technique."[20]

The other three mechanisms by which virtues become vices are: "when a change in the nature of the effects of a certain type of action transforms the character of that type of action"; "when a quality valued for its own sake is made available for sale"; and "a virtue may become a vice or simply a non-moral quality by a change in its relationship to a role which it partially defines."[21]

The Principle: Do Good and Avoid Evil: A substitution view also seems to be presupposed in the focus on virtues by the American Board of Internal Medicine (ABIM) in their sustained interest in establishing guidelines for "Assessing the Humanistic Qualities in the Internist."[22] This enterprise is based upon "the conviction that medicine has the moral significance of a calling. . . . that humanism is an essential part of internal medicine. Internists must function as personal physicians." (page 5) Specific virtues to be assessed are defined in the following principle:

Principle 1: The essential human qualities required of candidates seeking ABIM certification are integrity, respect, and compassion.
- Integrity is the personal commitment to be honest and trustworthy in evaluating and demonstrating one's own skills and abilities.
- Respect is the personal commitment to honor others' choices and rights regarding themselves and their medical care.
- Compassion is an appreciation that suffering and illness engender special needs for comfort and help without evoking excessive emotional involvement which could undermine professional responsibility for the patient.

The definition of compassion is especially interesting here. It is seen as linked clearly to "emotional involvement" which would make it spontaneous and natural, though what is recommended is the "golden mean" between callousness and such deep involvement that professional distance would be undermined. The other two traits listed are less directly linked to the emotions. They involve an enduring commitment to act in certain ways, but the motivational basis of this action is not specified.

Additional virtues are listed elsewhere in the ABIM report. For example, the subcommittee announces that it

supports an earlier task force's statement that the qualities a physician should possess if he or she is pursuing a career in internal medicine must include integrity, respect, compassion, honesty, trustworthiness, commitment and humility. (page 5)

Further, specific traits which are especially important in certain contexts are cited, as in principle 2.

Principle 2: Adaptive Relationships

+ The realities of institutional operations -- administrative policies, limited resources, and conflicting priorities between administration and house staff -- require sensitive, adaptive, and decisive behavior on the part of residents. They should establish and maintain honest and respectful relationships with supervisory faculty, consultants, peers, nurses, laboratory technicians, and other health-care personnel.

+ Residents may need to be reminded that patients and families deserve honesty, information, respect for the wishes of the patient, and fidelity to promises and commitments. (page 6)

In addition, the ABIM plans to undertake the task of developing ways to assess the presence of these traits. As a first step in this direction, they will include the category of "humanistic attributes" on the program director's evaluation form with descriptions of the extremes of the continuum dealing with "Personal Qualities and Interpersonal Skills in Patient Care." The negative extreme specifies "Lack of integrity, empathy, compassion, respect; insensitive, abuses trust, intolerant, unreliable; ineffective communication, poor rapport with family and patient." In the positive extreme, the physician "Always demonstrates integrity, empathy, compassion, and respect for patient; establishes trust; primary concern is for the patient's welfare; reliability; effective communication and excellent rapport with patient and family."

Needless to say, one who acts in certain ways from the motive of receiving an affirmative evaluation on this point would not truly possess the virtues in question.

The ABIM concedes frankly that there is a great deal of uncertainty in determining how these traits might be assessed and taught. They issue a challenge to both medical educators and medical ethicists to develop ways to achieve these goals. It would be worthwhile returning to the writings of John Dewey for some philosophical analysis of the problem of training and measuring such training for virtue.[23]

Other commentators list other virtues which ought to be promoted in physicians and patients too.

> A theory of virtue in medical ethics must explore that disposition most proper to the relationship between physician and patient -- trust.[24]

> "The Virtues of Good Physicians" include temperance, compassion, professional competence, courage, phronesis, justice, honesty.[25]

> Six responsibilities of professionals to clients are honesty, candor, competence, diligence, loyalty, and discretion.
> The three fundamental obligations of professionals to third parties are truthfulness, nonmaleficence, and fairness. Candor, with its requirement of full disclosure, does not pertain, because the professional does not have a special trust relationship to third parties.[26]

The American College of Physicians published an ethical code for physicians that also included some of the major responsibilities of patients. These latter included truthfulness and honesty, as well as compliance with the treatment plan developed.[27] A chapter of Pellegrino and Thomasma, *For the Patient's Good*, also includes a sketch of patient virtues.[28]

Equivalency Roles: Beauchamp and Childress[29] argue for a relationship of correspondence between principles of obligation and virtues. They offering a chart of equivalences, as shown in figure 4.

Fundamental principles	**Primary virtues**
Autonomy	Respect for autonomy
Nonmaleficence	Nonmalevolence
Beneficence	Benevolence
Justice	Justice or fairness
Derivative rules	**Secondary virtues**
Veracity	Truthfulness
Confidentiality	Confidentialness
Privacy	Respect for privacy
Fidelity	Faithfulness
Ideal actions	**Ideal virtues**
Forgiveness	Forgiveness
Beneficence (high risk)	Benevolence (high risk)
Acting mercifully	Mercy
Giving generously	Generosity

Figure 4

In contrast to this suggestion that virtues may be primary and fundamental, Beauchamp and McCullough[30] describe medical and professional virtues are derived from the two fundamental "models" of beneficence and autonomy:

> Beneficence -- Derivative Moral Virtues: From the principle of beneficence the physician's role-related virtues are also derived: truthfulness, trustworthiness, faithfulness, and the like.[31]

> Autonomy -- Derivative Moral Virtues: From the principle of respect for autonomy the physician's role-related virtues are also derived: respect, truthfulness, equanimity, faithfulness, and the like.[32]

Equivalency helps us see the meaning of the principle "Do Good and Avoid Evil." The principle cannot articulate in great detail what should count for good and evil. It must be directed further by the derivative moral virtues. These in turn have been formed from centuries of traditional values and teaching governing the proper relationship with patients under the general rubric of not harming them.

Franz Ingelfinger[33] insists that "arrogance" (by which he means an openly paternalistic benevolence) is a virtue; however, Carleton Chapman[34] cites this as one chief medical *vice* -- along with uncritical acceptance by practitioners of medical authorities.

Although Charles Fried focuses much of his description of the ideals for physician-patient relationships in terms of the deontic category of rights, he does seem to be getting at virtue notions when he describes the physician as "one whose professional activity is a personal expression of his own nature."[35]

Samuel Gorovitz offers a comprehensive list of "characteristics that I associate with the good physician":

- has and maintains a high level of technical competence, including both the knowledge and the skills appropriate to his specialty;
- is unfailingly thorough and meticulous in his approach to his specialty;
- is aware of the dependence of clinical medicine on medical research and equally aware of the experimental nature of clinical medicine;
- sees patients as persons with life stories, not merely as bodies with ailments;
- sees beyond simplistic slogans about health, nature, and life to the complexity involved in selecting goals for treatment;
- has a breadth of understanding that enables transcending the parochialism of his own specialty;
- understands his own values and motivation well enough to recognize that they can be in conflict with the patient's interests;
- is sensitive to the diversity of cultural, interpersonal, and moral considerations that can influence a patient's view of what is best, in process or outcome, in the context of medical care, and has the judgment to respect that diversity without undermining the integrity of his own moral commitments;
- has a respect for persons that shapes his interactions with patients, staff, and colleagues alike;
- has the humility to respect patient autonomy, the dedication to promote it through patient education, and the courage to override it when doing so seems justified;
- has the honesty to be truthful both with himself and with his patients about his own fallibility and that of his art; and
- has the sensitivity to recognize moral conflict where it exists, the motivation to face it where it is recognized, the understanding to consider it with intelligent reflection where it is faced, and the judgment to decide wisely following such consideration.

It is a tall order. But many physicians meet it, and more approximate to it reasonably well. The question is whether it is possible to increase the extent to which physicians on the whole are of this character.[36]

We have seen considerable variation in this chapter as to what a virtue is (i.e., the relative importance of affective versus cognitive dimensions and the relation between these), what role they properly play in medical ethics (and, in particular, whether they can ever function as a *substitute* for deontic principles), and just what traits are to be fostered. All the authors we have surveyed in this chapter would agree that some attention to motivation and to becoming a certain sort of person is important as a corrective to an exclusive focus in most medical ethics discussions on the right thing to do. If all physicians and all patients were to come to do "the right thing" on every occasion, but they did so on the basis of unworthy motives (e.g., fear of legal repercussions), then medical ethics will have been a failure. The ultimate goal of medical ethics teaching and scholarship is to foster individual moral development and moral relationships that incorporate the best human traits of character.

C. Strengths of the Virtue Model

First, as Jonsen and Hellegers point out, the stress on character, motives, and roles is compatible with the patterns of thought incorporated into codes of professional ethics -- which, in turn, influence the way professionals think about ethics. Thus, this approach is more likely to make immediate sense to practicing professionals than most (if not all) the other approaches we have examined. Indeed, no less notable and "mainstream" a moral philosopher than Prichard granted that virtue language was more engaging than the standard, deontic language of ethical theory:

> This sharp distinction of virtue and morality as coordinate and independent forms of goodness will explain a fact which otherwise it is difficult to account for. If we turn from books on Moral Philosophy to any vivid account of human life and action such as we find in Shakespeare, nothing strikes us more than the comparative remoteness of the discussions of moral philosophy from the facts of actual life. Is not this largely because, while moral philosophy has, quite rightly, concentrated its attention on the fact of obligation, in the case of many of those whom we admire most and whose lives are of the greatest interest, the sense of obligation, though it may be an important, is not a dominating factor in their lives?[37]

Second, a virtue more readily allows a focus on certain topics of obvious interest to those seriously concerned about morality -- for example, the importance of human feelings, the tragic nature of moral choices, the importance of the affective dimension of human relationships. For this reason, this approach is more likely than others to allow a place for emphasizing the importance of imaginative literature and affective exercises in the process of moral education and instruction. We need not go so far as Gorovitz's suggestion: "Why not require that each [medical] student spend a forty-eight-hour period in a hospital ward, in a bed, playing a patient role as a participant-observer of the full hospital day in the life of an inpatient?"[38] But the use of imaginative literature (which he also recommends) can be an important method of influencing the affective dimension of the relevant virtues.

Third, as both John Dewey[39] and Stanley Hauerwas[40] point out in somewhat different ways, a virtue approach provides the possibility of reconciling the age-old dichotomy between deontologism and teleologism in ethics.

At the level of ethical theory, these differences would remain as criteria for selection of which traits are to be admired and encouraged. For the extreme utilitarian, it would seem that the only fully admirable trait would be *benevolence*. Since promoting the general good is the one and only fundamental goal of the moral life, on this view, consistency demands that the highest admiration be reserved for those who make this their personal goal (i.e., for those who are motivated solely by benevolence). Similarly, a stringent Kantian would have to say that *conscientiousness* is the only morally admirable trait: "the first proposition of morality is that to have moral worth an action must be done from duty."[41] A virtue theorist might see that the only truly admirable moral trait is a *constant disposition to do good*, as we have discussed it throughout this chapter.

However, this having been said, there is still room for justification of other, more specific character traits on both teleological and deon-tological grounds -- even if these amount to somewhat of a compromise with the fundamental principles involved. Thus, Mill is consistent with the spirit of utilitarianism when he says that "in the long run the best proof of a good character is good actions"[42] and points out that utilitarians "resolutely refuse to consider any mental disposition as good of which the predominant tendency is to produce bad conduct."[43] In other words, the test as to which settled dispositions are to be considered virtues is to measure their *consequences*. Similarly, Beauchamp and Childress are consistent with the spirit of deontologism when they postulate the "primary virtue" of nonmalevolence corresponding to the deontic principle of nonmaleficence, the virtue of respect for autonomy corresponding to their principle of autonomy, and the virtue of justice or fairness corresponding to their principle of justice. A Rossian might also postulate primary virtues of fidelity, gratitude, self-improvement, and repentance corresponding to the remaining principles of Ross's basic list. In each case, the spirit of the deontic principle informs the settled trait of character.

But, although these differences in justification show up from "outside" the virtue, at the level of ethical theory they will not be noticed from "inside," by the person who embodies the trait. For him or her, the immediate motivating force is the emotion embodied in the virtue and not either a calculation of consequences or an allegiance to principles. The grateful person, for example, acts from immediate feelings of gratitude -- not from either a utilitarian calculation of the contribution of such actions to the general welfare or a Rossian direct insight into the moral bindingness of a principle of gratitude. The person who embodies the trait of gratitude acts because she *feels* grateful at the moment, or better, because she is disposed to be grateful. Thus, teleologists and deontologists would not differ within the framework of the specific virtues.

Finally, this viewpoint is not frightened by relativism and disagreements; and it may include resources which other approaches lack for reconciling these differences. A virtues approach is predominantly a recipe for individual and personal action. Because it is recognized that individual discerning judgment incorporates a complex of internal affective factors, we can tolerate variations in specific decisions. It is this trait that characterizes the thinking of Jonsen on casuistry to be discussed in the next chapter.[44] This approach is usually accompanied, as well, by a principle of nonjudgment: that it is morally inappropriate to judge the decisions others have made and that the only appropriate moral concern is developing and maintaining one's own character.

D. Weaknesses of the Virtue Model

First, it may be unrealistic to suppose that this approach will avoid or resolve moral disagreement. Since there is likely to be at least as much disagreement about the nature of "happiness" or "flourishing" as about ethical principles, there is still abundant room for moral disputes -- and there is no *a priori* reason to believe that disputes about ends will prove any more tractable than disputes about principles.

Second, as William Frankena has pointed out in his critical articles in *The Monist*[45] and *The Journal of Religious Ethics*,[46] in order for an ethics of virtue to serve as a guide to action, it must be supplemented by independent principles for action. This suggests that the *most* we can hope for from this approach is a complement to one of the other models we have examined, not a replacement for the others. This view is confirmed by the analyses of Beauchamp and Childress, Beauchamp and McCollough, and Jonsen, as we have seen.

Third, there is a danger inherent in approaching issues from this basis alone. It is all too natural to assume, from this perspective, that disagreements about what action is appropriate can only stem from deficiencies of character. Recently on surgery rounds a resident was thoroughly excoriated by an attending physician who called his moral character into question because of a clinical judgment he had made.

Fourth, there is the danger of confusing moral character with traits of professionalism. This is the mistake made, in our judgment, by H. Thomas Ballantine, Jr.,[47] in a recent lecture -- and, to a lesser extent, also made by Carleton Chapman[48] in an essay in the same issue of *The New England Journal of Medicine*. To suggest, as both authors do, that the responsibilities of a physician to render what Fried calls "personal care" to his or her patients arise from a "social contract" (Chapman) or principle of "noblesse oblige" (Ballantine) by which the society accords special economic and social status to physicians suggests this confusion, but Ballantine's attempt to extort the continuation of this status by threatening that physicians will no longer regard themselves as having these responsibilities if their privileged status is eroded makes it obvious that he is not appealing to a moral basis to ground the traits under discussion. In addition, many of the specific traits which are commonly included in such appeals, as well as in professional codes, embody what Chapman calls "guild rules and rules of etiquette governing the conduct between professionals" rather than moral elements *per se*.

Perhaps the most problematic of the consequences of a pure virtue approach to the resolution of issues is the way in which one person's "precept and example" become another's view of viciousness. Recall Ingelfinger's postulate of arrogance as an essential virtue and Chapman's view that it is the chief medical vice. Many physicians justify paternalism on the grounds of their role relationship. Yet an extreme form of this problem is revealed in the defense by Nazi commanders of violent and brutal acts or participants in the Iran/Contra affair on the grounds of the virtue of conscientiousness: "I was only doing my duty." Clearly, as the traditional theory of virtue itself required, motives and acts must be judged separately, and objectively. One does not act virtuously, despite the highest internal conscientiousness, when performing a bad act. An example of this analysis can be found in the virtue-theory rejection of euthanasia (seen as murder) even when the motives might be kindness or the avoidance of continued cruelty. It is much more difficult to act virtuously when conflicts among goods arise, as they do in medicine, than when the choice between good and evil is put before us.

E. Conclusion

Stressing the virtues is very important in a society of strangers. Patients always expect interior motivation towardsthe good in any health-care worker they encounter, even if they have never seen this person before. Further, as Stephen Toulmin indicates, such a stress on virtue provides for personalism, a rich understanding of complexity, and flexibility that an ethic of rules and policies simply cannot provide.[49]

Nonetheless, the trade-off for these qualities is a danger of capriciousness. There is an enormous variance among what persons regard as good acts, from child pornography to adoption, from assassination of world leaders, from holy wars and hostage taking to peace talks and mediation, from expanding military budgets to expanding health-care costs. This variance suggests the key ingredient of the virtue ethic that is lacking in a pluralistic society-coherent community values. After all it is these values that are to be instilled, interiorized in persons so that they become wise and prudential actors. Nonetheless, the medical profession can be viewed as such a community of coherent values. It makes these explicit in established relationships with patients so that there are commonly understood duties and roles. There is every reason to believe that the principle-virtue *nexus* discussed in these pages will bear much fruit in moral debates.

NOTES

1. Gregory E. Pence, Ph.D., *Ethical Options in Medicine* (Oradell, NJ: Medical Economics Company, 1980), p. 17.

2. Ibid., p. 202.

3. Albert R. Jonsen and André E. Hellegers, "Conceptual Foundations for an Ethics of Medical Care," in *Ethics and Health Care*, ed. Laurence Tancredi (Washington, DC: National Academy of Sciences, 1974), p. 8.

4. William K. Frankena, "Prichard and the Ethics of Virtue," *The Monist*, 54, no. 1 (1970), 1-17. Reprinted in *Perspectives on Morality: Essays of William K. Frankena* ed. Kenneth E. Goodpaster (Notre Dame, IN: University of Notre Dame Press, 1976), see especially pp. 150-151.

5. Ibid., p. 150.

6. Saint Thomas Aquinas, *Commentary on the Nicomachean Ethics*, trans. by C. I. Litzinger (Chicago: Regnery Press, 1964); *Summa Theologiae*, I,II (New York: McGraw-Hill, 1964).

7. Recall that Drs. Neil Barber and Thomas Nejdl were indicted for murder in California for withdrawing fluids and nutrition from a patient who suffered a brain trauma after elective surgery. See *Barber v. Superior Court*, 147 CA 3d 1006 (CA 1982); 195 Cal Rptr 484 (Dis Ct App 1983), 147 Cal App 3d 1054 (1983).

8. The American Medical Association Judicial Council, "Reports of the Judicial Council of the American Medical Association, December 1984," *Journal of the American Medical Association* 253 (April 26, 1985), 2424-2425.

9. Of course, this is the primary method for training children in the early stages of moral development. Here the trait to imitate is much admired. But it is expected that adults have transcended such imitation unless they find themselves in new and uncertain territory. In those circumstances as well they may adopt imitative models of moral conduct during their first days of training. See: Laurence Kohlberg, *The Philosophy of Moral Development* (New York: Harper & Row, 1981).

10. Graber, Beasley, Eaddy, *Ethical Analysis of Clinical Medicine*, p. 68. Emphasis added.

11. Henry K. Beecher, "Tentative Statement Outlining the Philosophy and Ethical Principles Governing the Conduct of Research on Human Beings at the Harvard Medical School," in *Experimentation with Human Beings*, ed. Jay Katz (New York: Russell Sage Foundation, 1972), p. 848.

12. Franz Ingelfinger, "Arrogance," *New England Journal of Medicine* 303, no. 26 (25 December 1980), 1507-1511.

13. See Thomas Aquinas, *Summa Theologiae*, IIa IIae, QQs. 47-170.

14. Preamble to "Ethical Principles of the American Medical Association (1847)," quoted in Jonsen and Hellegers, "Conceptual Foundations for an Ethics of Medical Care," p. 6.

15. Francis Peabody, "The Care of the Patient," *Journal of the American Medical Association* 88, no. 12 (19 March 1927), 877-882.

16. J. Graner, "The Primary Care Crisis: Part II: Physician as Laborer," *Humane Medicine* 3 (May 1987), 20-25.

17. Ibid., 22.

18. Pence, *Ethical Options in Medicine*, p. 199.

19. Alasdair MacIntyre, "How Virtues Become Vices: Values, Medicine and Social Context," pp. 97-111.

20. Ibid., p. 106.

21. Ibid., pp. 106-107.

22. American Board of Internal Medicine, "Evaluation of Humanistic Qualities in the Internist," *Annals of Internal Medicine* 99, no. 5 (December 1983), 720-724. See also Gregory Pence, "Can Compassion Be Taught?" *Journal of Medical Ethics* 9, no. 4 (December 1983), 189-191.

23. John Dewey, book cited at beginning of our text. Also the current thinking of Kohlberg, cited above, and others working in the field of moral development.

24. Jonsen and Hellegers, "Conceptual Foundations for an Ethics of Medical Care," 8. Cf. the redefinition of trust in Jay Katz, *The Silent World of Doctor and Patient* (New York: The Free Press, 1984).

25. Pence, pp. 202-211.

26. Michael D. Bayles, *Professional Ethics* (Belmont, CA: Wadsworth Publishing Company, 1981), pp. 86, 104.

27. Ad Hoc Committee on Medical Ethics, American College of Physicians, "American College of Physicians Ethics Manual," *Annals of Internal Medicine* 101, nos. 1 and 2 (1984), 129-137, 263-274.

28. Pellegrino and Thomasma, *For the Patient's Good*, chapter 9.

29. Beauchamp and Childress, *Principles of Biomedical Ethics* 2nd ed., pp. 265-266.

30. Beauchamp and McCullough, *Medical Ethics*.

31. Ibid., p. 40.

32. Ibid., p. 49.

33. Franz Ingelfinger, "Arrogance."

34. Carleton B. Chapman, *Physicians, Law, and Ethics* (New York: New York University Press, 1984), especially chapter 7 and Conclusion.

35. Charles Fried, "The Good of Personal Care," *Medical Experimentation* (Boston: American Elsevier, 1974), p. 77.

36. Samuel Gorovitz, *Doctors' Dilemmas: Moral Conflict and Medical Care* (New York: Macmillan, 1982), pp. 192-193.

37. H. A. Prichard, *Moral Obligation*, p. 12n. This footnote is the focus of discussion in Frankena, "Prichard and the Ethics of Virtue."

38. Gorovitz, *Doctors' Dilemmas*, p. 200.

39. John Dewey, *Theory of the Moral Life* (New York: Holt, Rinehart & Winston, 1960).

40. Stanley Hauerwas, *Vision and Virtue* (Notre Dame, IN: Fides Publishers, 1974).

41. Immanuel Kant, *Foundations of the Metaphysics of Morals*, p. 16.

42. John Stuart Mill, *Utilitarianism* (Indianapolis: Bobbs-Merrill / The Library of Liberal Arts, 1957), p. 26.

43. Ibid.

44. Albert Jonsen, "On Being a Casuist," in *Clinical Medical Ethics*, ed. Ackerman et al., pp. 117-130.

45. William K. Frankena, "Prichard and the Ethics of Virtue."

46. William K. Frankena, "The Ethics of Love Conceived as an Ethics of Virtue," *The Journal of Religious Ethics* 1 (Fall 1973), 21-36.

47.   Thomas Ballantine, Jr., "Annual Discourse -- The Crisis in Ethics, Anno Domini 1979," *New England Journal of Medicine* 301, no. 12 (20 September 1979), 634-638.

48.   Carleton B. Chapman, "On the Definition and Teaching of the Medical Ethic," *New England Journal of Medicine* 301, no. 12 (20 September 1979), 630-634.

49.   Stephen Toulmin, "The Tyranny of Principles"; see also David C. Thomasma, "The Possibility of a Normative Medical Ethics."

CHAPTER EIGHT
Towards a Unitary Theory
of Clinical Ethics

There is something fatally flawed about constructs of ethical reasoning and understandings of moral principles that fail to place principles in the realm of practice. The problem is familiar in the philosophy of science. Some persons argue that theories, like Darwin's about evolution through natural selection, or the theory of quantum mechanics, or the unified-field theory, lack explanatory power because they are too abstract and generalized. There is some truth to this claim, but it is simple minded as well. The reason is that principles cannot function at all unless they are applied to a situation in which boundary and other conditions instantiate the principle. Laws in science, or principles in ethics, cannot explain anything in isolation; but then they are not functioning as *principles* (i.e., as sources of inferences) when standing in isolation from application. Ethics, like medicine, is theory about practice. It arises from, and returns to, practice.[1]

Further, the rationalistic model of linear, step-by-step deduction or induction, is too narrow to do justice to the complexities of medical or ethical (indeed, any) decision-making. It is probably more nearly valid as a post factum or retrospective reconstruction of central argument reasoning, than a real reflection of the ongoing processes that occur during decision-making.

The rationalistic model has no current validity in either experimental research on decision-making (which demonstrates that persons make decisions largely intuitively -- including highly technical decisions by experts such as physicians)[2] or in the structure of scientific theory itself. Science and medicine do not proceed in linear, deductive fashion.[3] Even if, at one time, such processes did reflect the current understanding of scientific reasoning, and ethicists chose to imitate science as much as possible in forming their discipline, a new sort of unitary medical ethical theory is now called for.[4] This call is especially timely, given our more balanced understanding of scientific and medical reasoning today.

The task of constructing such a theory is enormous, but no more so than that faced by scientists attempting to construct a unified-field theory from so many conflicting data about subatomic particles. Put another way, medical ethics is not the only field where problems of theory and practice arise. Our task is aided by the analysis of strengths and weaknesses of the application, mediation, validation, determination, origination, and virtue models. There is no guarantee that the method we choose to analyze the theory/practice dilemma will ever resolve the deeper metaphysical questions of *praxis* and *theoria* and their relation. Our focus is less demanding than that. We wish, instead, to propose a practical model of bioethical hermeneutics that combines both theory and practice. Our greatest challenge will be to suggest ways in which conflicting approaches can cohabit in a unitary theory.

The rest of the chapter proceeds as follows. First, we discuss the way clinical ethics mediates between theory and practice in medical ethics. Then we explicate the medical basis of clinical ethics, a foundation that can provide for the creative cohabitation of frequently conflicting approaches. Next, we note some important features of the models studied which are to be avoided. Fourth, we catalogue the major features of the unified theory. Fifth, we sketch a biomedical hermeneutics needed to adjust and form clinical ethical judgment. We close with some general points about the relation of theory and practice in medical ethics.

A. Clinical Ethics

Why are the words "clinical ethics" in our title for this chapter? In our view, there are a number of branches of ethics in medicine. However, we are in search of guidelines that can be put to use in clinical decision-making by both physicians and patients. Our examination of ethical theories thus far has demonstrated that the clinical focus of medical ethics requires greater stress on the context than more general theories provide.[5]

Germane to our reasoning models is the challenge put to them by Franz Ingelfinger, the distinguished late editor of *The New England Journal of Medicine*. Ingelfinger charged that philosophers and theologians create a kind of absolutist ethic which cannot be employed in particular cases and is of little use to practicing physicians. He noted: "The practitioner appears to prefer the principles of individualism. As there are few atheists in fox holes, there tend to be few absolutists at the bedside."[6]

Both inductive models (validation and origination), for example, attempt a more careful "fit" between the realities of the medical setting, and of life itself, and the principles, rules, axioms, and theories of medical ethics. In fact, one of the results of our research into various reasoning models has been our discovery that thinkers such as Ramsey, McCormick, Veatch, and others employ several models of reasoning. This is not to say that generally deductive thinkers suddenly become predominately inductive ones. Indeed it is hard to imagine Veatch proceeding inductively or Siegler deductively. Rather, our point is that the kind of casuistry implied in Ingelfinger's observation about clinical judgment spills over into medical ethical reasoning as well.[7] This casuistry embodies an effort to fit various principles, axioms, rules, policies, guidelines for action, inductive products, and professional and personal virtues into a decision-making scheme along with patient, institutional, and social values.[8]

This requires an ethics that is a practical discipline. As Professor Peter Redpath notes, "Debates in ethics are so interminable today because contemporary ethicians, while maintaining some of the language of classical moral discourse, by and large, don't have the foggiest ideas what classical philosophers meant by a 'practical science.' A subject like ethics makes perfect sense in the teleological and scientific universe of Aristotle, but it is a mass of confusion in the mechanistic and post-enlightenment world of contemporary philosophy."[9] According to Redpath, individual moral acts are subjected to critique in order to apprehend the practical universal criterion that gives them their virtuous or vicious character. This practical universal helps a person synthesize values, choices, attitudes, and appetites.

As can be imagined, the agony patients must go through in reassessing values as they come to grips with serious illness requires that persons will make decisions on the basis of their own (perhaps fragmented and diverse) values rather than upon allegiance to one or another formally organized moral system or abstract principle. In their eventual decision the role of their particular, individual crisis will have led them to a different form of commitment to a principle, such as the principle of "preservation of life." Moral theory is thus "validated," but not in the way it is in other models. In clinical ethics reasoning, moral theory is existentially validated by individuals and (to some extent) societies working out their moral problems. Previous theories are radically altered by that process, and may even be rejected altogether.[10]

This personal process is not just a matter of arbitrarily rejecting cherished values. In some instances, a decision might be made that merely neglects fundamental values. For example, a couple normally opposed to abortion, might chose to obtain one, not because they reassessed their values, their fundamental moral theory, but because they ignored them in the mix, pressure, and drama of the present crisis. When they learn that the mother's health is threatened by continuing the pregnancy, nothing else enters their thinking but the urgent necessity of avoiding this threat. The consideration of the life of the fetus does not occur to them at this point. Or finding their situation overwhelmingly complex, they might have chosen not to decide, to do nothing and let nature take its course. Although to others this path looked like they had once again reaffirmed their commitment to life, and once again chose to preserve their anti-abortion beliefs, in fact they did not. The operative value is actually a sort of fatalism.

The point to be pressed is that the unitary theory we propose in this chapter will attempt to incorporate authentic features of existential (or clinical) decision-making in health care, and that primary among those features is both a place for standards (on the basis of which a critique of values takes place), and the practical realities that cause the crisis and feed into the standards themselves.

B. The Medical Basis of Clinical Ethics

In this section we will show that medical reasoning involves ethical thinking. At first blush, this claim may seem trivially true to many readers. However, much clinical diagnosis theory presents clinical reasoning as a purely technical matter--neglecting the value and ethical components of this process of judgment. By contrast, we shall show that both clinical diagnosis and therapeutics involve value judgments, some of which are ethical in nature. For this reason, it will be important to show how the theory/practice relationship in medical ethics actually derives from the theory/practice relation in medicine itself. Further, the medical basis of this relation provides the unitary ground of the clinical ethics theory we advance in the final section.

Recall that we claimed in previous chapters that (1) a merely deductive medical ethics would be inadequate because much more complex reasoning is required to resolve problems, and (2) medical ethics is not just applied normative ethics but also a branch of medicine itself (in the ways we carefully delineated it in chapters 5 and 6).

Both diagnosis and therapeutics involve values, however, values that may conflict among themselves or among others. Some of these values are ethical. As a result, decisions to be made must take all these values into account if medical ethics is to be properly understood.

As Erich Loewy writes: "Compassionate discretion is as necessary in the moral considerations of clinical problems as it is in technical ones. Moral and technical factors are inseparable elements of choice, demanding compassionate discretion if judgments are to be well made."[11]

The extremes to be avoided when discussing medical ethics are, on the one hand, the notion that medicine is a value-free science applied to individuals, and, on the other hand, that ethics is an externally valid discipline "brought into" the medical setting to resolve dilemmas. Somewhere between these two extremes lies the truth of the matter. Physicians often speak of a "therapeutic window" between too little and too much of treatment. Our claim is that there is a "philosophical window" as well, a window between too external a relation of medical ethics to medicine and too intimate a relation.

That medicine is not a value-free science can be seen from a consideration of its nature. Medicine can be defined as a relationship between a doctor and a patient.[12] It is neither "what doctors do," nor "what patients do" to stay healthy.[13] What doctors do is *not* just ruminate like scientific theorists and philosophers. When they do this, when they study and do research in the basic sciences, they are practicing (if the word can be used) the biological science they employ. When they practice medicine, by contrast, they apply *theory about practice* to individuals or to the community. Medicine, as distinct from the basic sciences it uses, is not theory about how the body works (that is physiology), but theory about how to work *with* the body to bring about desired outcomes. Since these outcomes are valued, by medicine as a discipline and by patients for the therapeutic benefits they bring, they are goods towards which the physician-patient relation aims.[14] As such, they may constitute, under specific circumstances, normative ethical guidelines for that relationship.[15]

Furthermore, as Engelhardt has argued, even diagnostic categories of disease are value-laden, just as are "clinical indicators" by which one arrives at a diagnosis.[16] Thus, concepts of health and disease, used as the theory about practice in medicine, themselves represent values the patient, hospital, and/or society may accept or disregard, consider significant or insignificant, judge too risky or worth the risk. For example, "alcoholic," once a sanitized term to displace the moral disapproval found in the term "drunkard," has now itself sometimes become a term signifying a moral evil. In this way a whole complex of values requiring ethical analysis and judgment come into play in every medical judgment. Raymond Duff and Jurrit Bergsma suggested a schema of value clashes between patient and physician, physician and other physicians, physicians within themselves, and between both patient and physician and society on the macro, micro, and meso levels.[17] From this consideration, one may calculate an almost infinite series of important to less important ethical issues arising from each medical transaction.

Similarly medicine is not just the activity of keeping healthy, eating right, exercising, taking vitamins, going on vacation, or other health-related activities that persons may do on their own for their own well-being. These activities do not qualify to establish a relationship with a physician. One has no "suffering" (*pati*) to bring to the attention of a physician. Further, one may even suffer but choose to deal with the problem on one's own -- a minor burn, for example. Then one becomes one's own physician. The discipline of medicine is not perceived as needed. Not having sought a professional's help, one is not really a patient.[18]

The ideal object of the doctor-patient relationship is healing or health, if healing is understood broadly to include compassion, care, and restoration of personal self-reliance.[19] Since healing is a moral activity, and an analysis, either explicit or implicit, of values in that relationship of healing is required to reach decisions (medical judgments as to what is good for patients), the "right and good" decisions are inherently moral ones. That is to say, medical judgments are ethical when reflectively based on values in the relationship and on moral principles and axioms which bear on the relationship.[20]

Ethics is involved in the doctor-patient relationship even when no tremendous moral quandary exists.[21] Ethical analysis of the decisions contemplated or made in the doctor-patient relation is characteristically a second-order function of medicine itself, rather than an application of ethical theory to yet another practice. In other words, if the moral character arises from medicine's own *praxis*, then at least a portion of ethical analysis is based on the *praxis* and not on applying independent theories to it, as if the latter were like decorative icing on the cake of medicine. Consequently, medical ethics should not be seen as a "foreign" discipline invited into and potentially resented by medical practice. Instead it should be a reflective function of medicine itself.

An important objection to this thesis needs to be raised. The objection is that medicine cannot expect answers from philosophy. Hence, there can be no real use in developing a clinical ethics, since it could not rest on well-established principles. This point was formulated by Alasdair MacIntyre.[22] The objection can be phrased in a stronger form: If we are to have a deductive ethics, then we must be able to deduce applications from generally agreed-upon moral principles. Because in a pluralistic age there are no ultimate moral universal principles, one cannot look to philosophy, applied ethics, or even medical ethics for any genuine help in resolving moral quandaries in medicine.[23]

The answer to this objection can take two forms. The first would be a defense of deductive ethics in a pluralistic age. The defense would argue from the horrible social consequences of living in an ethically rudderless society. This approach is apologetic rather than substantive however. The reason is that general principles offered for our universal acclaim have failed to gain it. Thus, Charles Fried's efforts to argue for an objective standard, a libertarian position in health care distribution, can easily be contrasted with Robert Veatch's contract theory (that would exempt a practitioner from the obligations of social justice to care for individuals), and both of those would markedly contrast with the Rawlsian notions of Norman Daniels.[24] Unfortunately, the universal principles of ethics have never been as universal as their advocates claim they ought to be.

A second approach to responding to the objection is to be preferred. In it one answers MacIntyre's objection by agreeing that a deductive ethic, and hence any notion of applied ethics, is fatally flawed. In its place can be substituted some alternative form -- such as the ethics of discretion proposed by Stephen Toulmin.[25] Although the general character of this mode of ethical analysis is clear, its outline has yet to be filled in:

A) A purely deductive ethic, or applied ethics, fails to recognize that ethics cannot have the degree of certitude enjoyed even by the physical sciences. At best, ethics can only be morally certain, that is, a certitude ranging from generally speaking true, for the most part true, to rarely if ever true.

B) General principles are important, for they free us from the tyranny of culturally-driven habits, but they must be fitted together with middle level principles or axioms that arise in part from medicine's own goals in trying to resolve both cases and social policy.

C) The source of some of these axioms might be a practice itself, as MacIntyre now argues.[26] The development of excellence in a practice (such as medicine) can be part of these axioms, provided we recognize the moral nature of the practice.

D) Axioms in medicine are agreed upon by most medical ethicists and clinicians.[27] A list of generally held axioms would include: Do no harm, Relieve suffering, Tell the truth (especially about dying to dying patients), Obtain informed consent, Help establish personal wellbeing, and Respect the dignity of human life independent of the status of the person. These axioms arise from the goal of medicine to heal. It makes no sense to harm, for example, if one aims at healing. The moral character of these axioms rests on the value of healing as an ethical act itself.

E) Skepticism about the validity of applied ethics, such as Kai Nielsen's,[28] is well-placed if aimed at general principles, but not if aimed at the consensus about middle-level axioms. However, one does not go about resolving ethical dilemmas by applying principles to situations. Rather, efforts are made, like those of the Roman Catholic casuists of old, to respect as fully as possible all the many normative factors competing in the case. One does not stamp a case with one principle, just as medicine does not solve a diagnostic problem in this way. Instead, a whole host of factors is considered through hypothesis formation, and decisions are made according to analogy with other cases. The analogue may be an ideal or classic pattern of disease, a series of inductive cases reviewed seriatim, or even a combination of the two. Similarly, the ethical dilemma is resolved using analogical reasoning. In each case or policy dilemma, one may call on a number of principles and axioms to help bring about a resolution.

F)   In this view, medical ethics is just as much a branch of medicine as it is a branch of ethics. We do not "apply" principles as much as "ferret out" resolutions.[29]

Consider the role of the ethics consultant as a "practice" of medical ethics. Bringing the skills and language of ethics to medicine does not certify the ethicist as an expert in moral judgment, nor does this qualify him or her for health professional roles.   The most effective role of the ethicist is that of a consultant who makes recommendations based on the literature and disciplines of ethics and medical ethics.[30]

The claim that a clinical consultant role is legitimate, but must be distinguished from that of a moral expert, bears some further examination, as it will shed light on the distinction between the two for clinical ethics.   Nielsen's problem with applied ethics is that no ethicist has the expertise to make recommendations. But a concern about avoiding what can be called moral posturing is common to all ethicists, including those, like Robert Veatch, who do hold that a normative medical ethics is possible.[31] Yet Veatch holds that medical ethicist may be consulted by physicians or even by patients regarding specific ethical advice.[32]   Further he recognizes that a particular ethicist may be in a position of representing a community of belief or even a community of principles that he or she may confidently interpret.   Such a position may be held by a rabbi, minister, or priest trained in ethics, just as the priests in the Karen Ann Quinlan case and Robert Brophy case represented both family and church values against the effort by health professionals, hospitals, and other churchmen to keep these patients on life-support systems. One might imagine that an ethicist could also conceivably make recommendations in the context of a community of doctors and patients sharing values of secular humanism.

The nub of this point, however, is that a position of moral expert must be distinct from a position of consultant making recommendations.   On the one hand the moral expert would be one who could tell the moral rightness or wrongness of an action from some criterion known, promulgated, and acknowledged by all.   On the other hand, a consultant would be one trained in a discipline that has bearing on a case, voluntarily asked to recommend a course of action or several courses of action to the persons morally responsible for making a decision, and held responsible for the quality of prudential judgment. This distinction is not subtle. The moral expert represents bigotry, if the principle upon which the recommendation is based is not, indeed, universally recognized or held. A philosopher in pretense of moral expertise would irremediably violate any expectations for control of *hubris*. By contrast, a consultant is a person admittedly functioning within the conditions of prudential or practical, fallible judgment. One of the conditions of such judgment is to consult others with wisdom and experience about the affair at hand.

But, one might ask, is not the distinction between judging right from wrong (the moral expert) and making recommendations (the medical ethics consultant) just begging the question? Is not what Nielsen and many others object to the very act of making recommendations? Is not this act one which assumes one knows the right thing to do? If so, how does this differ from moral posturing?

The answer to these questions now depends on one's philosophy of medicine and the role of medical ethics within it. If one views medicine as a science independent of application to human beings, any ethical considerations are regarded as external to this "value-free" enterprise. In making a recommendation, one would be "applying" an external discipline, ethics, to an unrelated one, medicine. The recommendation would therefore have to stand or fall for its validity on ethical principles and the coherence of its reasoning. We have just seen that the universality of these principles is in doubt. Further, they are so contentless that their meaning is almost wholly derived from interpretation; the latter is certainly subject to capriciousness or arbitrariness. Hence, to make an ethical recommendation on this model of medicine is an objectionable enterprise, unless the physician, patient, and ethicist all share a common belief in certain principles and interpretations, say at Oral Roberts University Medical Center. But even religious faith today lacks the monolithic character necessary to carry off such a program.

Contrariwise, if one views medical ethics as a branch of applied ethics, and the latter as a branch of deductive ethics, then a similar otiose identification of making recommendations with moral posturing occurs. Again in order to justify one's recommendations, one must rely on a criteriology based on a defense of universal moral principles and/or the rightness or wrongness of an act based on these principles. The same difficulties apply in this view as they do in the medicine-as-science view.

However, recommendations are not the same type of action as judging the moral right and wrong of a course of action if one sees that medicine is a relationship between health care professional and patient. In this relation decisions made are based on values inherent in that relationship, as well as external ones from the institutional and social context. Further, decisions are made based on indicated courses of action, not commands. In this model, then, the medical ethicist need not blush when called an expert. He or she must know the literature, must know ethics and philosophy, must know sufficient medicine to be informed about the moral crunch in the case, and *most importantly*, must know analogous cases. The recommendation is therefore based on a community of values, some shared and some not, in the practice -- that is, in the relationship of healing. Second, it is based on analogous cases. Third, it is based on an objective of respecting a set of normative values in the case. Thus, the moral right or wrong according to abstract theory is not at issue. What is at issue is a moral rightness *in accord with the standards of practice*-- in this instance, the axioms of medicine, respect for patient values, and the like.

Whether it is right or wrong to withhold intravenous fluids from a dying patient, as two physicians did in California, is a subject of endless debate in the sphere of theoretical and applied ethics.[33] In an ethics of analogical reasoning, the question is not an ethical judgment of this kind. Instead it is: Does such an action conform to standards of practice (where these standards include value-components as well as technical judgments)?

To illustrate this, take an example from family practice medicine. As one of us (Graber) has argued with John Eaddy, "family care" is a moral norm of family practice medicine.[34] What does this mean for the resolution of cases? Suppose a young teen-aged girl asks a family physician for a prescription for birth-control pills.[35] Normally an ethicist would be tempted to resolve this case by applying to it external principles of confidentiality, truthtelling, and autonomy. To do so, however, is to neglect the real ethical drama for both the patient and the physician. It is this: the physician has a commitment to treat the patient in the context of family relationships. Whether or not the physician knows the family intimately as friends or colleagues, socially, or hardly at all, the physician's commitment to the family functions as an axiom of practice: treat each person so as to strengthen family wellbeing.

Clearly, to accede to the girl's wishes without taking family unity into account (even though this axiom may later be rejected in the resolution), would be to violate the clinical ethics of family medicine. This point holds true irrespective of the conclusions one might draw from the principle of autonomy -- that the minor has reached the discretionary age and that her wishes must be respected, or from the principle of confidentiality -- that the discussion with her can never be revealed to others, particularly to her parents. Naturally, one would try to respect all the normative factors in the case as fully as possible -- for example, by suggesting to the patient a family discussion on the issue of sexual activity. But, in the last analysis, a family practice physician could not violate the axiom of his or her practice by prescribing the pills without some measure of parental accession or some effort to reach a family consensus on the problem the teenager presents.[36]

C. Things to Avoid

In constructing a unitary theory of clinical ethics there are some important things to avoid. Although our list is not exhaustive, it is derived from the lessons learned from the weaknesses of the models we have discussed in the previous chapters. (See Appendix B for a summary.)

1. Formalism

First, the theory should not neglect the circumstances of moral crisis to such an extent that the principles formulated become so abstract that they have no inherent power to apply to the realities of life. Most persons live their lives on the basis of moral precepts learned from their parents or churches. "My mother always told me to forgive and forget." "My father always said that you will never regret kindnesses to others." Although these precepts are not ethical principles, they contain enough moral content that they are reasonably able to guide personal choices.

We are not arguing that all moral principles should be prescriptive. Rather, we argue that they contain enough moral content derived from various sources that they can overcome the objections made in chapters 2 and 3 to the application and mediation models. Put another way, ethical principles like Respect for Persons, or Respect for Autonomy, should be seen, not merely as conditions of possibility for moral discourse and as such, meta-ethical formal principles, but as two of a number of normative guides for action.

2. Absolutism

The second feature of past ethical theories to avoid is absolutism. Most likely this feature entered ethical theory in imitation of science during the Enlightenment. Just as in science one attempted to reach abstract, general laws of the universe, so too ethicists attempted to reach the same level of certitude in ethics. This was certainly Kant's intent, i.e., to construct a sufficiently rigorous practical science, a metaphysics of morals, that would be immune to the encroachments of new scientific discoveries.[37]

For Kant, ethical statements are not inductive, nor can they be conditional on the basis of experience. Yet, as Dewey noted in 1928, Kantian notions of overweening obligation and duty are simply not appropriate in circumstances in which the element of uncertainty is so powerful.[38] In virtually all medical ethics cases, the most striking feature is the uncertainty about outcomes. For a couple whose fetus has ambiguous genitalia, not knowing the sexuality of the fetus, the degree of retardation that might accompany this condition, and the eventual procreative possibilities closed off for their unborn child, establishes a crisis they face about their values. No single duty or obligation can function on an *a priori* basis in fashioning their decision about aborting a "defective" fetus.

Ethics was not always as rigorous as the Enlightenment required. Although Aristotle, and St. Thomas following him, did try to construct a science of ethics, their perception of the nature of a practical science differed from later constructs, as we noted earlier. In particular, no principle in practical affairs was capable of obtaining mathematical or metaphysical certainty. Rather the certitude in ethics, precisely because of its practical nature and the ever-changing quality of human life, could only be *ut in pluribus*, to use Aquinas' phrase, "generally, for the most part true."[39]

Of course, current conceptions of science have advanced far beyond the those of the ancient Greeks and Middle Ages. But they have also advanced beyond the Enlightenment during which Kant worked, and the pre-nuclear, industrial age of Mill. Our ethical theory should embrace, instead of outdated notions of absolutism, a more probabilistic certitude comparable to that found in modern scientific theory. We call this type of certitude, "conditional," meaning that when certain conditions exist, a probability of x exists that value A will be judged more important than value B because of the applicability of principle P over P'. Thus, there is a high probability that patient autonomy ought to be respected in primary care settings (the condition) because the value of autonomy (A) generally precedes that of other competing values like paternalism (B) because the condition of primary care medicine where the problem may not be serious and the patient's judgment not impaired will allow the principle of autonomy (P) to apply more appropriately than other principles like beneficence (P').

3. Atemporality
The third feature of past ethical theories to eliminate is atemporality. This feature was closely allied to the effort to establish general principles that would apply beyond particular circumstances. Although this is a laudable goal, a more sophisticated understanding of complex decision-making suggests that a clinical ethics theory would provide for at least a distinction between long- and short-term perspectives. Just as Adam Smith employed the image of an invisible hand guiding the marketplace, so too is there an invisible hand guiding our complex society. As a consequence it is impossible for anyone to understand completely the consequences of their own actions. Actions taken in the short-term may have a long-term consequence that is unforeseen. For this reason unabashed consequentialism is inherently flawed. It may appear that an action is good in the short-term, but it may turn out badly in the long run.

A good example of the short-term, long-term dynamic can be found in the case of Baby M. Baby M's father, William Stern, a scientist, engaged a surrogate mother because he and his wife judged it unwise to have a child. Mrs. Stern suffered from a mild case of multiple sclerosis, and being a physician on the faculty of Albert Einstein School of Medicine, she was concerned that a pregnancy would exacerbate her condition. She would risk serious health impairments and possible paralysis. Mr. Stern offered $10,000 to a woman who accepted his sperm through artificial insemination nine times until she conceived and eventually bore the baby. The baby's case became prominent when Elizabeth Whitehead, the surrogate mother, refused to give up the baby on the grounds that she had formed a bond with it. In reaching a decision, Judge Harvey Sorkow of the New Jersey court that heard the case argued, among other things, that since men had some time past been allowed to sell their sperm, the same right to sell one's womb could not now be denied to women.[40]

Regardless of the faulty parallelism involved (it should have run from sperm to egg, not sperm to womb), the fact that another human being is now involved (rather than just sperm or egg), and the question of whether Whitehead's womb was sold or merely rented, it seems clear at this point that if society had foreseen the avenues for potential abuse which follows from its approval of "selling" reproductive tissue, it might have been more cautious about permitting males to sell sperm in the first place.[41] If short-term expedient is not checked by long-term thought (the struggle about theoretical issues), then precedent-setting arguments like that of the New Jersey court judge would continue unabated. The "is" of practice would become the "ought" (or at least the "permissible") of morality.

Long-term thought must necessarily be more abstract, conceptual, and critical than short-term thinking. It must critically examine theories, principles, precepts, and axioms in our decision-making. These frameworks of cultural mores are subject to intense scrutiny in the existential crisis of each clinical dilemma. But there must also be short-term thinking. By contrast to long-term, short-term thinking is characterized by analysis, casuistry, and realism. This kind of thinking has been especially lacking in public policy formulations about health care.[42]

D. Major Features of a Unitary Theory

The major features of a Unitary Theory of Clinical Ethics follow from the strengths of the models we have examined in the book. (See Appendix B for a summary of Strengths and Weaknesses.)

1. The Virtuous Character of the Principals

No amount of theory, principles, or guidelines will suffice if individuals and institutions do not possess professional and personal virtues. This requirement extends to patients as well.[43] Among key professional virtues are benevolence, respecting the wishes of patients, truthtelling, promise-keeping, prudential judgment about the proportion between intervention and outcome, and dedication to the preservation of life.[44]

Among the virtues required of patients are truthtelling, promise-keeping, compliance, and trust.[45] The physician, in order to bring about the good for the patient, must know many facts about the patient and hold that patient's trust, not the least so that the patient's compliance with the agreed-upon (and sometimes--as in recovery from heart attacks or managing chronic diseases like diabetes--imposed) regimen will be extensive.

A good example of the moral mayhem that results when physicians do not appear to follow accepted behaviors (we call them virtue-expectancies) can be found in the story of Robert Oldham, M.D., a fellow of the American College of Physicians, and a distinguished cancer researcher and clinician. Tiring of the endless guidelines, politics, and bureaucratic delays required by the "government-academic system" as he calls it, Oldham left his post at the National Institutes of Health (NIH) where he was founder and director of the National Cancer Institute's Biological Response Modifiers Program for four years. He then opened his own corporation in Franklin, Tennessee, calling it "Biotherapeutics," where for a fee (reportedly $19,400 plus the cost of a month-long hospitalization), patients can receive bio-therapy for cancer (predominately Interleukin 2). This reception bypasses the waiting lists at the six university centers that now offer this experimental therapy.

Many physicians argue against this for-profit corporation to dispense still-unproven therapy even while acknowledging that Dr. Oldham is no quack peddling apricot pits. But he clearly has departed from standard virtue-expectancies among physicians. As he acknowledges, few physicians send him their patients. But, ironically, many physicians or members of their families themselves are his patients.

Objections to Oldham's corporation reveal hidden violations of expected virtues. These are now listed as "vices" with the objector's name at the end:

a) Taking the discoveries of others without working in the system (Robert Gallo of the NIH's NCI discovered Interleukin 2 in 1976). (Dr. DeVita)

b) Using for profit a discovery generated at public expense (Dr. Relman, editor of the *New England Journal of Medicine*).[46]

c) Using a methodology not based on logical progression from scientifically sound information we now possess (Dr. Greco).

d) Employing a kind of scientific prematurity for using and selling experimental treatment to patients.

e) Acting "too far out on a limb."

f) Employing a theory of the "uniqueness of cancer cells" that is "a lot of baloney." (Dr. Chabner) (The therapy in this reference using monoclonal antibodies reputedly costs $35,000 per patient).

g) Using research therapy as a moneymaker without contributing to overall research aims. This is "cynical" (Dr. Relman).

h) Making patients pay for the costs of experimental therapy as yet unproven (Dr. Goldie).

i) Performing actions not up to the standards of the medical community, "which is not lily-white to start with" (Dr. Preston).

j) Being unjust: "I find it morally offensive that this treatment is available only to those with large sums to pay for it" (Dr. Relman).[47]

Almost all of these objections, except for the questions about payments, can also be raised against physicians, like Dr. Leonard Bailey, who transplanted the baboon heart into Baby Fae,[48] or more tellingly, against charlatans themselves.

From the list of negative traits or vices, it is possible to generate the virtue-expectancies of physicians involved in experimental treatment. They would be:

a) Employs the discoveries of others by working within the established medical-academic system.

b) Never charging for profit for a treatment generated at public expense.

c) Employing a logically sound and consistent scientific methodology.

d) Never offering to patients for sale a treatment that is yet unproven.

e) Always acting within the boundaries of established standards.

f) Employing only those theories that make sense to most other researchers.

g) If charges are to be made for experimental therapy, the amounts received must be returned to the research effort.

h) Being just by offering therapy to all, regardless of ability to pay.

Whether or not individual physicians follow these virtues, it is instructive to see the idealism of modern medical research practice revealed in them.

A similar kind of moral mayhem ensues when patients violate the virtues expected of them. When patients knowingly lie to physicians or destroy the trust required by the relation between them, they not only potentially hurt themselves (by lying about not having pains in the chest, for example), but also they destroy the relationship's purpose. Two examples demonstrate this side of the virtue equation in the doctor-patient relation.

The first example was the case of Chad Green. Recall that Chad Green was an infant who contracted leukemia. His parents brought him to a treatment center on the East Coast, but Chad suffered a relapse. Although the infant's physician felt that therapy against the relapse was medically indicated, the parents protested. They would not agree with such therapy. The physician reluctantly agreed, since the boy presumably suffered the relapse while still on initial induction chemotherapy. But the patients had lied to the physician. They had not been giving the boy his medication on schedule, thus betraying the trust in the relationship in favor of other values that remained confused throughout this case. Once this lie became apparent to the physician, he sought a court order to treat the boy on the grounds of child abuse. The parents fled the state, eventually going to Mexico to obtain unproven therapy. The boy died there.[49]

In this case, the lie to the physician created a breakdown in trust as well as to a distortion of clinical reasoning such that any chance of healing Chad was destroyed. Violated, then, were the virtue-expectancies that:

a) Parents have the best interests of their child always in mind. (Here there would be a dispute, because the parents held that that is precisely the motive of their actions).

b) Patients and guardians tell the truth.

c) Patients and guardians trust the physician.

d) Patients and guardians trust modern medical research modalities.

e) Patients and guardians fulfill moral commitments to heal by cooperating with the academic research community, the same community Dr. Oldham rejected in setting up his private corporation.

A second example comes from California. There Elizabeth Bouvia, a 28-year-old woman, entered a hospital with the express intention of committing suicide. She had been married, had a miscarriage, and was abandoned by her husband after her diseases became too difficult to manage. She suffered from cerebral palsy so badly that she could now only lift her head slightly and move a few fingers. Her situation was complicated by severe, painful arthritis, requiring morphine delivered through a chest tube. This controlled but did not eliminate the pain.

Since she was bedridden, she had to rely on others to provide for all her needs, including feeding and "toileting," as the California Appeals court so delicately called it. She could not, then, accomplish her suicide on her own without great suffering; thus, her entrance into a hospital for help from physicians so she could die painlessly. They, and the hospital administration, refused. When she tried to starve herself to death, they introduced a feeding tube in her nose against her consent.

A lower court agreed with the moral commitments of the doctors and the hospital to preserving life, although it was ruled that the hospital must discharge her if she chose to go somewhere else to die. This she did, setting up her death watch in a motel, where staff from the hospital came by to look after her medical needs. After a few days of this, Elizabeth agreed to return home and to eat again. Later she returned to another hospital where her bed became a moral and legal battleground regarding assisted suicide. An Appeals Court (and the Supreme Court of California by its refusal to hear the case) held that Elizabeth had the right to determine her own treatment, and that the doctors and hospital must help her in what is now called "assisted suicide."[50]

This is a very complicated case. But it reveals the difficulties that arise when patients depart from what we have called the virtue-expectancies. Bouvia's request violates major duties and commitments (virtues) of both physicians and hospitals. The Court decision in her favor requires a new moral theory of medicine whose value outlines are only now becoming clear. As Joseph Fletcher argues, physicians should have as a virtue, a commitment to help people attain a "smooth death." The axioms to be respected in such a theory would be the right of the patient to determine his or her own treatment, and the new virtue itself, now expressed as a willingness to assist in suicide under rigidly controlled conditions.[51]

As alternates to this view G. H. Stollerman suggests that the doctor-patient relationship is still an unequal one (in terms of expertise) and that, on a case-by-case basis, doctors must still be permitted to assess the quality of the patient's judgment.[52] This theory is similar to that implied in the actions of the Chad Green physician, who judged that the family's judgment about the best interests of the child was impaired. One of us (Thomasma) has argued that a different sort of theory can emerge from the Bouvia case. According to this theory, physicians may still be able to retain the virtue of commitment to the preservation of life while balancing that with the duty not to prolong dying. This balance is called "death induction." By this is meant constructing a therapeutic plan for a dignified death by employing techniques of withholding or withdrawing therapies (passive euthanasia techniques).[53]

The elements of the virtue theory describe only the characteristics, habitual modes of acting for the good, of the principal players in the clinical dilemma. The commitments we can expect from virtuous character are not always appropriate, otherwise no one would break out of the expected modes of action; nothing new would be tried; the boundaries of medical research, practice, and delivery would remain rigidly circumscribed.   Nonetheless they do provide a foil to empty formalism in medical ethics.   Much more is needed than virtue precisely because of the weaknesses we noted about the virtue theory itself.

2. Ranking of Values

Clinical   medical ethics is largely played out in the arena of middle-level axioms and moral rules. For this reason we argued that absolutism is to be avoided in drafting a general theory. Decisions are made in a real-time frame. Cases are like dramas, or films. New concerns arise each day, each moment. As a consequence, the axioms or norms examined in this book are shuffled to fit the circumstances, just as one employs different tools when designing and constructing a cabinet. Methods of resolution are like those tools -- they are chosen for their "fit" to the task at hand.

When, for example, a discussion occurs between two residents on different services regarding the allocation of a bed in the Intensive Care Unit, a number of norms come into play. One resident, on the oncology service, knows that shortly a patient will be brought in by her husband. She has disseminated breast cancer in the bones, liver, and brain. As recently as the last month, she has been hospitalized for stabilization of her electrolytes, re-hydration, and pain control. There is a Do Not Resuscitate Order in her chart. The problem is that each time she is treated, she is able to return home. No one can say when her final admission will be, but it surely will come soon. The second resident is on the surgical service. She has a patient, the town alcoholic and drug abuser, who has recently been operated on for an intestinal blockage, and now suffers from post-operative gangrene in some of the tissues of the abdomen.   He, too, is in a life-threatening condition.

The norms that arise in these cases are the preservation of life, providing high quality medical care to patients who need it, responsibly managing one's case, and respecting the wishes of the patients to be treated or not to be treated.   A typical principle involved in these cases is beneficence, acting in the best interests of patients; a correlative axiom (which includes a motif of personal care) might be phrased as: *act to maximize the benefit of one's particular patient*.   The allocation of the single bed available must be made on the basis of one or another of these norms, axioms, and the values they represent.

When choices must be made like this one, it becomes clear that the "fit" between the axioms and values, and the case, must include an additional factor that assists in the process of ranking values. In this case that factor might be a consideration of the authentic purpose of the Intensive Care Unit. Although both patients need intensive care, the surgical patient more closely fits the purposes of the unit, since he has a chance to recover and return to his life, however abnormal. Intensive Care Units are not intended to be locations for treating the dying patient. For this reason, even Do Not Resuscitate Orders and other attempts to limit treatment are difficult for the staff to comprehend there and to manage properly. Such a consideration, then, might lead to a decision in favor of the surgical patient. One value basis of the decision would be that respect for patient determination will less likely occur in the ICU for the cancer patient, than in a regular room or medium care environment. A second value principle might be that when allocating between two worthy candidates for intensive care, preference should be given to the patient that has the best chance for long-term survival.

Our purpose was not to suggest the only way to resolve the conflict between the two residents, but to illustrate how a Unitary Theory of Clinical Ethics must include a provision for the ranking of values. This ranking takes place by appeal to at least two sources: first the purposes and realities of the clinical setting involved, and second, the values considered more important in the individual cases. Respect for patient decision-making and long-term survival were two such values illustrated. These considerations would change from case to case, instance to instance within cases, and environment to environment. Incidentally, this is the reason why the virtue or character of the individuals or institutions involved becomes important as well. For this character imbues the care taken about the values involved, the thoroughness by which they are examined, as well as the compassion and commitments one must take for granted in the discussion.

3. The Role of Theories and Principles

In the previous section of the chapter, we argued that atemporality was to be avoided. In its place principles and theories should be seen as establishing boundaries for conduct, and carving out the prescripts of conscience that must guide societies, institutions, and individuals in decision-making. To use the earlier example of selling (or, more properly, renting) one's womb, the level of theory and principle requires a thorough analysis of this practice. Once it is established that one may or may not sell one's womb for profit, a guideline is established by a theory of "ownership of one's body" for surrogate motherhood. By extension, the principle of ownership can then apply to other bodily organs; it may be proposed, for example, as the fundamental principle in a theory of organ retrieval, whereby organs might be put up for sale to the highest bidder.[54]

That was a public policy example. The feature of clinical ethics that stands out most prominently is what Loewy calls "the uncertainty of certainty."[55] What he means by this is that all actions impose on the actor a requirement to remain flexible and to accept fallibility. There is no absolute certainty in clinical ethics, and in clinical judgment.

In fact, we argued in the previous section that absolutism must be avoided because only conditional certitude can be found in ethics. The process of hypothesis formation in medicine and in clinical ethics (the former about the diagnosis and treatment, the later about the primacy of certain values over others in the case) relies upon sorting and sifting probabilities, outcomes, likelihoods, and similar notions. A bad result may occur from this reasoning. Pusillanimity would be a vice of both physicians and clinical ethicists.[56] Risk is an inherent property of all human choices.

We will show how a Unified Clinical Ethics Theory can incorporate elements of the virtue, deontological, and consequentialist theories of ethics in a realistic and pragmatic nexus. The method used to resolve a particular case is often a function of the questions that case raises. Non-formal responses to the dilemma, responses such as, "Dr. J. is a good doc, so I can support what he does," or "She had the patient's best interests at heart," are mixed with more formal elements. Virtues of the participants are checked by arguments about a hierarchy of values in this particular case, and arguments about rules (interpretants) of middle-level axioms.

All of these are set within a social and cultural context by appeal to theory, particularly to theories about the role individual persons and their values ought to play in determining the social good, and what kind of society ought to emerge from the technico-practical interventions medicine can make into personal and social life.

E. Biomedical Hermeneutics

To this point, we have argued that a unitary theory of clinical ethics must rely on the virtues of the interpreter(s) of the crisis situation and deontological guidelines for the conscience of the interpreter(s). In medicine those guidelines are provided by the moral nature of the enterprise itself, by the social and cultural mores, as well as by applications of more general ethical theory. Nonetheless it is the interpreter(s) who must do the applying, mediation, determination, validation, and origination not only about the decisions but also about the inductive and deductive products of which we spoke in earlier chapters. Just as in modern scientific theory the role of the observer has received critical attention, so too should it in medical ethics.[57]

Lodged in virtues and principles are goods developed from social experience. These goods guide arguments and decisions. In medicine, life itself forms the basis of the goods, but there are two conflicting interpretations of the value of life in medicine -- the sanctity of life and the quality of life.[58]   There exists no central consensus in the community about the proper weight to be given either of these interpretations of the value of human life.

In place of such a consensus, medicine must aim at meaning. In a "meaning-centered medicine," as Barnard has called it, meaning is "a process of imagining and maintaining dependable structures of order and significance in life."[59]   We take this to mean that the object of medicine is to restore and maintain as far as possible the ability of persons to pursue their values, purposive striving.   Thus a process of negotiation about values is required to reach the proper interpretation of the good of life that lies at the center of medicine.   Thus Barnard argues that the primary clinical behavior of medical practice ought to be enhancing the "mutual participation by doctor and patient in the construction of meaning for, and assignment of value to, the successive moments of the illness experience."[60]   Medical hermeneutics is a bilateral process.

At this juncture, the relation of interpreting events to ethical theory becomes clear.   Viewed from the point of view of goods, each ethical theory can be seen as a "hermeneutic of the good."   Alan Donagan, for example, argues that Aquinas' first principle stems from a loyalty to personal goods.   He formulates it as: "Act so that the fundamental human goods, whether in your person or in that of another, are promoted as may be possible, and under no circumstances violated."[61]   The principle implies Kant's respect for persons as well as the practical goods of such persons, their perfections, not just abstractions.   Medicine must serve the purposefulness of human life. Health is a condition of possibility for the pursuit of values (goods) that transcend the physical life alone.   Thus, the interpretive principle of medicine, based on the value of human life, offers a weighting of the quality of life (properly negotiated) over the sanctity of life.   James Walter states in this regard: "When medicine cannot any longer promote this goal [purposiveness] for a patient at all, or when, by its interventions, medicine will place a patient in a condition that makes the pursuit of purposefulness too burdensome, then medicine has reached its limits *on the basis of its own principal reason for existence*" (author's emphasis).[62]

Thus, to return to mutual negotiation about values in medicine, interpretation is required because, as Boyle puts it, "There is more to the obligation to love someone than to that of respecting his or her humanity."[63]   Interpreting the good in the situation is also required. It is not just a matter of good clinical behavior.   It is also ethically mandated.

We now explore the process of interpretation in medical ethics, or as it should properly be called, biomedical hermeneutics.

1) A Statement of the Unitary Theory

Recall the statement made under the conditional certitude section. It can now be expanded to encompass a summary statement of the Unitary Theory:

> *Certain conditions (C) are present in this case such that the probability (x) exists that Value (V) A will be judged more important than B by (I) interpreters because the Principle (P) p' will more likely apply to the case than p".*

The rest of this section is an explication of this theory.

2) Conditions

The conditions of a case are its context. We have argued that the context functions as a moral rule. Contexts function as interpretative precepts that guide the process of weighing values and balancing competing principles and axioms. A primary care context, as we noted, would require emphasis on patient self-help, the wellbeing the family, and patient autonomy in general, all other things being equal. A tertiary care context, by contrast, such as that found in emergency medicine, requires emphasis on interventionist medicine, an assumption in favor of treatment unless otherwise noted, and even necessary medical paternalism. Hence, the first important factor to discern in a medical ethics case is the context. Some examples of interpretant contexts follow.

    2.1) The State of Medical Capability.--The state of our advances in medical knowledge, technology, technical skills, and the resulting capabilities in managing disease entities play an enormous role in interpreting values, principles, axioms, and rules, and assigning weights to them.

For example, traditional means of determining death have developed on the basis of two central values: (a) respect for life, and (b) respect for persons. These were clothed in the common view of the human person as comprised of body and soul. They were also shaped by the technological possibilities for extending life in critical illness (in the past, these were virtually non-existent). Thus when the central processes within the body ceased, this was taken to mean that the dissolution of the human person had irreversibly taken place.

Empirical criteria for irreversible dissolution developed on the basis of this understanding: detecting no pulse, hearing no heartbeat, noticing that no condensation appeared on a mirror when held to the mouth or nose.

If a patient is admitted with these symptoms to an African bush hospital, she may still be considered dead today, even though we have more sophisticated "brain-death" criteria. In the absence of the technology to restore and maintain vital functions, the older criteria suffice.

2.2) Medical Indications. -- The context also determines the medical indications to be employed in reaching decisions for treatment. If a person is dying in an oncology ward of a tertiary care university hospital, it may be judged medically indicated by the health professionals caring for the patient to offer a new, as yet unproven therapy, that might just "buy a few more months of life." Patient acceptance of death might then be counterbalanced by perspectives that draw significantly upon experimental medicine. The patient may thus be encouraged not to give up yet. This would be especially appropriate if the patient acceptance of death had been arrived at only reluctantly -- by a patient whose value history includes a strong will to live.

But if that same person were dying at home under hospice care, there would be no experimental, "push back the boundaries" interpretative context. Rather the context would be one of comfort care, not pushing against the boundaries of survival. Medically indicated treatments in a hospice program are quite different than in a tertiary care setting. The decision to enter the context of hospice influences future decisions.

2.3) The Stratum of Care. -- Actually, each stratum of health care, primary, secondary, and tertiary, influence the relative weights one would give to patient autonomy, self-determination, medical interventions, even the role of the family.

Using the last as an example, in primary care, the family's judgment about what the patient should do rarely enters the decision. Usually, the physician and the patient together work out the therapeutic plan. Often it is no more dramatic than taking an antibiotic for 10 days, or lowering one's weight through diet and exercise. In secondary care, let us say after a heart attack, the family's perceptions and judgments come into play to a greater degree than in primary care. The husband will necessarily become involved in the wife's rehabilitation diet and exercise. The values of home cooking, the nature of a family meal, the way the family recreated will now be changed. Their previous values will also lead to adjustments in the ideal therapeutic plan. In tertiary care, during a diabetic crisis, the family may now have to articulate the values of the patient (who is now confused and very ill) in a way they have never before been asked to do. These values will help determine the application of a technology (like kidney dialysis) to the patient's life.

    2.4) Responsibility in Relationships. -- Just as the context changes through strata of care, so too do the responsibilities of those who care for the patient in these different environments. Thus the context of personal relationships give rise to moral responsibilities.[64]

3) The Existence of the Probability Factor

The probability factor (x) is the likelihood that certain values and certain principles will prevail over others in the case. In some cases the interpreters will see almost immediately that paternalism will necessarily prevail. Examples of such cases would be those in which small children are involved, or persons who have never been able, by reason of illness or mental disease, to articulate their own wishes. In other cases, it will be almost immediately obvious that the patient's wishes should predominate, such as when patients have expressed their wishes in legally executed and recognized documents like Living Wills, Advance Directives, or have appointed a durable power of attorney.

    The difficult cases are those in which the likelihood of some values and principles predominating over others is difficult to discern, either because of the complexities of the case or disagreements among the interpreters.

4) The Interpreters

All cases require extensive human engagement. The fundamental engagement of the physicians and patients, families, surrogates, hospitals, and social agencies (such as Child Welfare Agencies, or the Medicare referral process), is to interpret the case and the values involved. A foundation of internalized virtues is required for this important feature of every case. Even if absolutely every minute detail of every possible case could be spelled out on a computer and all cases fed into it for resolution, we would need to rely on the veracity and responsibility of those who performed these tasks for the computer. As it is, interpreters are involved in much more profound ways in analyzing the case and balancing its important features. The virtues spelled out in our chapter on virtue theory are all essential for the unitary theory to work properly.

    Thus, when children are being treated, it is not always the case that paternalism would predominate. In the case of a sixteen-year-old girl who refuses therapy for religious reasons, the interpreters must work with the realities of a sixteen-year-old's faith.[65] Respect for that reality is an important part of such a case, though it might not be in another case, say, when the teenager has just recently converted to a new faith, or when the teen expresses doubts about the validity of the faith. In other words, the particularities of the context change the way the interpreters view the predominance of some values and principles over others. We must be able to trust that they do this responsibly, and hold them accountable if they do not.

5) Values

There are two forms of interpretation at the level of values that articulate the hermeneutical activity of the interpreters. We call these forms *axiomatic* (or *intrinsic*) and *nomian* (or *extrinsic*).

5.1) Axiomatic. -- When the physician abruptly arrives at a catastrophic diagnosis, many medical ethicists consider it obvious that the principle of respect for persons dictates telling the patient "the whole truth," straight-out.[66] But this is far from clear-cut. In the first place, what does "respect for persons" mean in this context? To tell them may be regarded as acknowledging their rational capacities by inviting them to take part in the deliberations and decisions that must now be made.   Presumably, this is one central component of the notion of "respect for persons." On the other hand, it can hardly be considered a sign of respect to presume an unrealistic assessment of the patient's coping abilities and thus to overtax these in a way that will lead to a sense of humiliation and despair on their part. This example shows that the meaning of the principle of respect for persons must be carefully and constructively discerned in the process of applying it to a particular person.

This type of interpretation deals with the *content* of principles, developing their implications for substantive action-related matters through the medium of values. It is a value to understand respect as a kind of protection from harm rather than (another value) as straight-out truth telling.   Thus (following the same order as the principles cited above -- to which they relate), examples of axiomatic interpretation (value statements) would be:

»   Enhancing patient autonomy is an essential element of respecting persons (deontological).

»   Calculating the greatest good for the greatest number of people is a necessary component of enhancing the benefit of all (utilitarian).

»   The good in the case at hand is to restore the patient's sense of self-worth (natural law/virtue theory).

Of course, these are only three of innumerable axioms that can assist us in refining and specifying the content of principles. Once stated as bearing upon the case at hand, the interpreter also balances them, either consciously or unconsciously prioritizing them on the basis of their importance for the case.

One mistake of the application model was to overlook the

importance of middle-level axioms.   Adherents of that model view these as following from the fundamental principle in a mechanical, deductive fashion with the aid of (too often unexamined) minor premises.   In reality, the step from principle to axiom requires a creative process of construction and/or insight that is not adequately captured in the casual introduction of a minor premise in a syllogism. The practical effect of the application theorists' misunderstanding on this point was the wooden and uncreative interpretations of key principles that brought on the charge of "legalism" and "rule-worship" against them.

The mediation model tends to share the same mistake in both directions: (a) to trivialize the creative insight required for derivation of axioms from principles, and also (b) to assume that once these middle-level norms have been derived and stated, the remainder of the process of application to specific, concrete situations is a mechanical, deductive step.   Further creative interpretations (nomian interp-retations as well) are required.

The mistake of the validation model was to fail to recognize the role principles do play in guiding the process of discerning middle-level norms.   Axioms are concrete expressions of the "spirit" or "deeper meaning" of principles as well as the values of patients, physicians, hospitals, society, and culture.   Thus experience and context also make a significant contribution to the development of axioms; but they are also shaped in a fundamental way by principles.

Both the elements drawn out in the example about truth telling above can be understood as components of respect for persons.   There is another type of interpretation operative in reaching a specific norm for such a situation.   To this we now turn.

5.2) *Nomian Interpretation.* -- Given the intrinsic interp-retations that have been discerned in the truth-telling situation, we have nonetheless not yet been able to reach a point of a clear directive for action.   The problem now is that we have two *conflicting* directives: (a) to tell the patient in order to enhance autonomy through participation in decision-making, and (b) *not* to tell straight-out in order to preserve the patient's coping mechanisms.   What is now required is a discernment about which of these ought to take priority in a given case.   This is the form of interpretation we call "nomian" or "extrinsic" interpretation.   No less than the previous form, it involves creative insight or discernment.   Once again this discernment cannot be replaced by some mechanical deductive step.

General statements of priorities among the various axioms and the values they represent as they bear upon a specific case we have called "rules."   It is these that are derived from frameworks of interpretation that earlier we called "contexts."

An example of such a rule that might be used to prioritize among axioms in the truth telling case might be "First, do no harm." This rule is recognizable as a primary and essential norm of medical practice. Because of the context of medical practice, then, the axiom protecting the patient's coping mechanisms would predominate over the axiom of involving the patient until the patient was ready for the second axiom. Thus, application of the nonmaleficence priority rule would lead to a counsel not to tell the patient right now about the catastrophic illness. Instead, as a strategy to promote wholistic autonomy over the long run, it would be advisable to present the information to the patient gradually, in measured doses, accompanied by efforts to help the patient deal with the immediate emotional impact of each dose of truth. In this way, the coping mechanism can be strengthened to the point of acceptance of the whole truth. When this is accomplished, the objective of involving the patient in the decisions to be made can then be pursued.[67]

It is especially important to note how the nomian interpretation is influenced by the interpreters' assessment of the status of the patient's abilities. In another case in which those abilities to cope were not so fragile, the opposite weights would be given to the two competing axioms under the same rule.

6) Principles

Principles express norms for action at the most general level. Examples of principles we have examined are:

▸   Persons ought to be treated with respect (a deontological principle, one expression of Kant's second formulation of the categorical imperative).

▸   The benefit of all is a greater good than the benefit of a few (one fundamental presupposition of utilitarianism, a tenet some have called the principle of "universalism").

▸   One ought to do good and avoid evil (a basic tenet of the natural law/virtue theory).

Because these theoretical judgments are so general, however, there is still a large gap to be bridged in order to bring them to bear on specific concrete actions. As we saw in chapters 3 and 4, principles cannot be applied to concrete actions in the sort of straightforward, deductive manner proposed in either the application or mediation model. Instead they require processes of interpretation in the two ways noted above, to relate them to specific concrete actions.

The likelihood of p' taking precedence or p" in any case, then, depends on the context, the interpreters, and the axiomatic and nomian interpretations involving values.

7) Classification of Action Guides

It is important to recognize that action guides are classified variously as principles, axioms, and rules, not on the basis of their content, but strictly on the basis of their epistemic status within the system of thought. Thus the same action guide that functions as a principle in one system (e.g., the principle of respect for persons in a Kantian deontology) may serve as an axiom or rule in another (e.g., in a form of rule-utilitarianism in which it is discerned as the working guide to maximize the general welfare).

F. Conclusion: Theory and Practice

Theory and practice in medical ethics are heavily intertwined. Clinical ethics arises from and returns to practice. But just as importantly the theories, principles, and axioms of clinical ethics impinge upon current and future practice. Were this not the case, we would not have the following two worries: the practice worry and the theoretical worry.

1) The Practice Worry

The practice worry is most commonly found in the domino theory of moral decay. But it is also found whenever new mores creep into the standards of the day. According to this worry, current and new practices are inaugurated by the willful minority who flout accepted morality. These practices later become accepted by a majority of (largely unreflective) citizens. They are accepted as moral goods, or morally neutral activities, precisely on the grounds that they are present among the activities of society. There is no critical re-examination of values before the practices are introduced. Among current bioethical "worries" are abortion, euthanasia, treatment of defective newborns, surrogate mothers, genetic research on newly conceived beings, and withholding food and water from dying patients.

What is interesting about these worries from our point of view is the often dramatic (and correct) perception of the power of practice to lead to new moral theories that tend to establish the validity of the practice.

2) The Theoretical Worry

We do not often pay much attention to a comparable set of worries about theory. For those who introduce new practices, old moral theory is seen as a block, an outdated indoctrination of the masses, that impedes new practices (theories are sometimes precisely that). Consider the couple in the discussion of ambiguous genitalia cited earlier. Their religious conviction prohibiting abortion effectively blocks this avenue in their resolution of their dilemma. They must expend an enormous amount of psychological and moral effort with the principle of preserving life that blocks the solution of aborting the fetus.

Those who have accepted new practices sometimes do so after a thorough analysis of values (it is not as uncritical a process as the practice-worriers think). Most people must be concerned about the principles of conduct in any crisis situation when cherished values conflict. Worrying about principles, then, becomes a major part of human life -- the subject of numerous articles, books, pamphlets, editorials, and television specials.

In the unified theory, practice both utilizes and limits theory, and theory constantly checks and balances practice. Whether or not our particular brand of clinical-ethics theory is defensible (as we think it is), any description of medical ethics must include the components we have uncovered and discussed in this book.

In support of a diminished role for principles, it is important to realize that there are no unmediated truths. Principles themselves represent ought-statements that embody social consensus, as we noted in the first chapter. There is no Platonic ideal or authentic moral person or persons. All theory arises from practical problems and is constantly tested for its validity through social consensus. This social consensus is derived from past experience of individuals and the community. Even those who argue for principled moral behavior, that being ethical means acting on principle, must agree that such principles are mediated through the context of the current situation, and tested somehow for validity, even if that validity is no more than unbridled application to the new situation. At the very least, dilemmas in medicine arise when such principles come in conflict (whether with each other or with prior urgings of conscience) in individual instances. A minimal task of medical ethics is to fix the boundaries of such principles. Thus, interpreting the fit between situation and principles is an essential part of making moral judgments. It is a form of biomedical hermeneutics.

A principled ethic degenerates into rule worship unless it is rooted in -- and constantly checked against -- faithfulness to underlying values. Even Kant, the patron saint of legalism, acknowledged in the second formulation of the categorical imperative the rootedness of duty in esteem for humanity. Furthermore, these deep values may be represented in institutional structures as well as in abstract principles. One important point of attention to the "founding fathers" (or mothers) of institutions is to make the values embedded in the institution imaginatively vivid through accounts (often amounting to hagiography) of the personality of the founding figure.

The reason inductive models of ethical reasoning work, then, is that they can be as faithful to the goods embodied in structures and practices, in individual loyalties to a center of value, as the deductive models were faithful to the goods and values embodied in principles and axioms. In chapter 6 we uncovered the importance of "backdrop" for purely inductive models. The backdrop, recall, was an implicit assumption about practices (such as the importance of beneficence and negotiation in the doctor-patient relationship). It is now clear that the backdrop contained hidden value loyalties. It functions in inductive models as a center of values. Similarly, in chapter 7 we discussed the importance of fidelity or conscientiousness to a set of values. These virtues also contain the goods of human life. Hence, a complex of loyalties to the good can produce value-derivations that form the basis of bioethical decisions: conscientiousness about principles and axioms, fidelity to the values embodied in contexts, individual value histories, and negotiation.

Notes

1. Erich Loewy, *Ethical Dilemmas in Modern Medicine* (Lewiston: Edwin Mellen Press, 1986), pp. 19-32. Howard Brody states: "Medical ethics, after all, is supposed to be a guide to action; and our high-sounding ethical theories and methods will look unimpressive if they do not, in the end, offer practical guidance in the sometimes confusing world of medicine." *Ethical Decisions in Medicine*, 2nd ed. (Boston: Little, Brown, 1986), p. 35.

2. "Their decisions may be perfectly on the mark, but the way they arrive at them is certainly not in the rational mode," Robin Hogarth, University of Chicago Director of the Center for Decision Research, as quoted in Lynn Emmerman, "Decisions, Decisions," *Chicago Tribune* (10 April 1987), Section 5, 2. Center researchers have found, according to this article, that the more important a decision is to us, the less rationally we react. Values and attitudes play a complex role in making decisions. Although quantitative assessment of values and attitudes of patients towardsdecisions in medicine are potentially helpful, they remain problematic. See: H. A. Llewellyn-Thomas, H. J. Sutherland, A. Ciampi, J. Etezadi-Amoli, N. Boyd, and J. Till, "The Assessment of Values in Laryngeal Cancer: Reliability of Measurement Methods," *Journal of Chronic Disease* 37 (1984), 283-291; H. Llewellyn-Thomas, H. Sutherland, R. Tibshirani, A. Ciampi, J. Till, and N. Boyd, "Describing Health States: Methodological Issues in Obtaining Values for Health States," *Medical Care* 22 (June 1984), 543-552; H. Llewellyn-Thomas, H. Sutherland, R. Tibshirani, A. Ciampi, J. Till, and N. Boyd, "The Measurement of Patients' Values in Medicine," *Medical Decision Making* 2 (1982), 449-462; H. J. Sutherland, H. A. Llewellyn-Thomas, N. Boyd, and J. E. Till, "Attitudes Towards Quality of Survival: The Concept of 'Maximal Endurable Time,'" *Medical Decision Making* 2 (1982), 229-309; J. E. Till, "Quality-of-Life Assessment: Beware the Tyranny of the Majority," *Humane Medicine* 2 (1986), 100-104.

The complexity of decision-making also influences reasons why patients choose specific therapies or enter experimental therapy at all. See in this regard: A. M. C. O'Connor, N. Boyd, D. L. Fritchler, Y. Kriukov, H. Sutherland, and J. E. Till, "Eliciting Preferences for Alternative Cancer Drug Treatments: The Influence of Framing, Medium, and Rater Variables," *Medical Decision Making* 5 (1985), 453-463.

Decision-analysis methods hold promise for structuring ethical decisions as well. These result in highly complex and refined case analyses much as that done by James Vaupel, "Structuring an Ethical Decision Dilemma," *Soundings* 58 (Winter 1975), 506-524; also see David C. Thomasma, "Decision Making and Decision-Analysis: Beneficence in Medicine," *Journal of Critical Care* 3, no. 2 (June 1988).

3. Instead they proceed in analogical reasoning modes. See David C. Thomasma, "Philosophical Reflections on a Rational Treatment Plan," *Journal of Medicine and Philosophy*.

4. See, in this regard, Stanley Hauerwas, "Authority and the Profession of Medicine," in *Responsibility in Health Care*, ed. George Agich (Boston: D. Reidel, 1982), pp. 83-104; *A Community of Character* (Notre Dame, IN:

University of Notre Dame Press, 1981).
        5. Jonsen, Siegler, Winslade, *Clinical Ethics*, 2nd ed. 1986.
        6. Franz J. Ingelfinger, "Bedside Ethics for the Hopeless Case," *New England Journal of Medicine* 289, no. 17 (25 October 1973), 914-915.
        7. David C. Thomasma, "Philosophical Reflections on a Rational Treatment Plan"; Donnie J. Self, "An Analysis of the Structure of Justification."
        8. Albert Jonsen, "On Being a Casuist," in *Clinical Medical Ethics: Exploration and Assessment*. Ed. Ackerman et al., pp. 117-130.
        9. P. Redpath, "The Method of Moral Reasoning," *Contemporary Philosophy* 11 (15 February 1986), 2-4.
        10. Modern Roman Catholic moralists have spent a great deal of effort during the period after the Second World War adjusting their traditional teleological theories within modern categories such as mixed consequentialism, mixed deontologism, mixed deontologism of agency, and the like. This effort demonstrates the necessity of combining older theories with respect for the case itself.   See Thomas Ulshafter,   "Jacques Maritain as a Mixed Deontological Ethicist of Agency," *Modern Schoolman* 57 (1980), 199-211. From the point of view of casuistry, efforts have been made to reconsider the formal structure of moral norms and the role of good results in moral judgment. See Richard A. McCormick, "Notes on Moral Theology: 1976," *Theological Studies* 38 (1977), 57-114.   Thus the relative strengths and weaknesses of theory and practice are weighed with respect to moral thought. The overall result, as Lisa Cahill notes, is to distinguish Catholic moral thought from utilitarianism, even though this approach still "assigns an important role to consequences in moral judgment":   Lisa S. Cahill, "Teleology, Utilitarianism, and Christian Ethics," *Theological Studies* 42, no. 4 (December 1981), 601-629. Also see Charles Curran, "Utilitarianism and Contemporary Moral Theology: Situating the Debates," *Louvain Studies* 6 (1977), 115-156.
        11. Loewy, *Ethical Dilemmas in Modern Medicine*, p. 25.
        12. Pellegrino and Thomasma, *A Philosophical Basis of Medical Practice*, chapter 2; Graber, Beasley, Eaddy, *Ethical Analysis of Clinical Medicine*, pp. 14-17, 118-119.
        13. Cf. Pellegrino and Thomasma, "Response to Our Commentators."
        14. Thomasma, and Pellegrino, "The Philosophy of Medicine as the Basis of Medical Ethics." Also see Leon Kass, "The End of Medicine and the Pursuit of Health," in *Toward a More Natural Science* (New York: The Free Press, 1985), pp. 157-186.
        15. David C. Thomasma, "The Possibility of a Normative Medical Ethics." Also see Leon Kass, "Professing Medically: the Place of Ethics in Defining Medicine, " *Journal of the American Medical Association* 249 (13 March 1983), 1305-1310;   David C. Thomasma, "What Does Medicine Contribute to Ethics?" *Theoretical Medicine* 5, no. 3 (October 1984), 267-277; Graber, Beasley, Eaddy, *Ethical Analysis of Clinical Medicine*, pp. 118ff.
        16. H. Tristram Engelhardt, Jr., "The Concepts of Health and Disease," in *Evaluation and Explanation*, ed. H. Tristram Engelhardt, Jr., and Stuart Spicker (Dordrecht/Boston: D. Reidel, 1975), pp. 125-142.
        17. Jurrit Bergsma, and Raymond Duff, "A Model for Examining Values and Decision Making in the Patient-Doctor Relationship"; also see Jurrit

Bergsma, "Towards a Concept of Shared Autonomy," *Theoretical Medicine* 5, no. 3 (October 1984), 325-331.

18.   Edmund D. Pellegrino, "Toward a Reconstruction of Medical Morality: The Primacy of the Act of Profession and the Fact of Illness," *Journal of Medicine and Philosophy* 4, no. 1 (March 1970), 32-56; Edmund D. Pellegrino, "Being Ill and Being Healed: Some Reflections on the Grounding of Medical Morality," *Bulletin of the New York Academy of Medicine* 57, no. 11 (January-February 1981), 70-79; Graber, Beasley, Eaddy, *Ethical Analysis of Clinical Medicine*, pp. 11-14.

19.   Bergsma with Thomasma, *Health Care: Its Psychosocial Dimensions.*

20.   An interesting clue to this intersection can be found in Sheehan et al., who used a Kohlberg-based measurement test (The Rest Defining Issues Test) to demonstrate that the greater a resident's clinical judgment skills, the higher he or she scored on the Kohlberg scale of moral development. See L. Sheehan et al., "Moral Judgment as Predictor of Clinical Performance," *Evaluation and the Health Professions* 3 (1980), 393-404.

21.   Everyday ethical issues arising in medical practice, rather than dramatic ones, can be found as prompts for self-evaluation of physicians in Graber, Beasley, and Eaddy, *Ethical Analysis of Clinical Medicine*.

22.   Alasdair MacIntyre, "How Virtues Become Vices."

23.   Alasdair MacIntyre, "Why Is the Search for the Foundations of Ethics So Frustrating?"

24.   Charles Fried, *Right and Wrong*;   Robert Veatch, *A Theory of Medical Ethics*, pp. 324-330;   Norman Daniels, *Just Health Care*.

25.   Stephen Toulmin, "The Tyranny of Principles."

26.   Alasdair MacIntyre, *After Virtue.*

27.   See Beauchamp and Childress, *Principles of Biomedical Ethics*; Albert R. Jonsen, "A Concord in Medical Ethics," *Annals of Internal Medicine* 99 (August 1983), 263.

28.   Kai Nielsen, "On Being Skeptical About Applied Ethics," in *Clinical Medical Ethics*, ed. Ackerman et al., pp. 95-116.

29.   Charles H. Reynolds, John A. Eaddy, Karen K. Swander, "On Bridging the Theory/Practice Gap in Training Medical Ethicists," in *Clinical Medical Ethics*, ed. Ackerman et al.,   pp. 43-58.   When philosophers and physicians train students and fellows in clinical ethics in the clinical setting, their purpose is to resist their natural tendency to bring their favorite principle to bear on a problem. Instead educators want them to gain a new sense or discerning judgment about the role of *praxis* in developing not only the resolution but a new theory. (Howard Brody, "Teaching Clinical Ethics: Models for Consideration," in *Clinical Medical Ethics*, ed. Ackerman et al., pp. 31-42.)   All such students leave the training period with a heavy dose of reality-immersion.   All agree that this dramatically changes, even at times reverses, the way they think about problems, and the means sought to resolve them. (Glenn C. Graber, "Teaching Medical Ethics in the Clinical Setting: Objectives, Strategies, Qualifications," in *Clinical Medical Ethics*, ed. Ackerman, et al., pp. 1-30.)

30.   Donnie Self and Joy Skeel, "Potential Roles of the Medical Ethicist in the Clinical Setting," *Theoretical Medicine* 7, no. 1 (February 1986), 33-40; Howard Brody, "Teaching Clinical Ethics: Models for Consideration," in

Clinical Medical Ethics, ed. Ackerman, et al., pp. 38-39.

31. Robert Veatch, *A Theory of Medical Ethics.*

32. Robert Veatch, "The Medical Ethicist as Agent for the Patient," in *Clinical Medical Ethics*, ed. Ackerman et al., pp. 59-67.

33.   See Kenneth Micetich, Patricia H. Steinecker, and David C. Thomasma, "Are Intravenous Fluids and Nutrition Morally Required for a Comatose Dying Cancer Patient?"; David C. Thomasma, Kenneth Micetich, and Patricia H. Steinecker, "Continuance of Nutritional Therapy in the Dying Patient," *Critical Care Clinics* 2, no. 1 (January 1986), 61-70; J. Paris and Richard McCormick, "The Catholic Tradition on the Use of Nutrition and Fluids," *America* 156, no. 17 (5 May 1987), 356-361.

34.   Glenn C. Graber and John A. Eaddy, "Teens and Birth Control," in *Medical Ethics: A Guide for Health Professionals*, ed. John F. Monagle and David C. Thomasma (Rockville, MD: Aspen Publishers, Inc., 1988), pp. 73-89.

35.   This case forms the basis of a chapter of David C. Thomasma, *Medical Ethics: A Case Studies Approach*, a textbook published privately for the medical students at Loyola University of Chicago Medical Center, 1988.

36.   See Pellegrino and Thomasma, *A Philosophical Basis*, chapter 8.

37.   Immanuel Kant, *Foundations of the Metaphysics of Morals.*

38.   John Dewey, *Theory of the Moral Life.*

39.   Germain Grisez, "The First Principle of Practical Reason." Samuel Gorovitz and Alasdair MacIntyre acknowledge the same point in their "Toward a Theory of Medical Fallibility," *Journal of Medicine and Philosophy* 1, no. 1 (March 1976), 51-71.

40.   *In the Matter of Baby M, a Pseudonym for an Actual Person*, Docket No. FM-25314-86E, Bergen County, NJ.

41.   Baby M. court case.

42.   For example, individual cases exist where prudential clinical judgment saved lives despite bureaucratic obstanancy. Daniel, an eight-year-old boy, needed an operation to repair his eye after he was accidentally shot in the eye with shotgun pellets. His family were members of an HMO offered by the trucking company where his father, John Bohnen, worked.   Mrs. Bohnen received a telephone call from the HMO minutes before she was to take Daniel in for the operation to repair his right eye. The HMO's business office wanted Daniel to be seen by one of its medical consultants before he had the operation.   Mary Jane Bohnen told the HMO office that Daniel's surgeon warned that any delay might cost the boy his sight. The HMO still insisted.   The referral physician quickly confirmed the need for the operation. By the time this verification ensued, however, it was too late to save his vision in that eye; see: M. L. Millenson, "Health-Care Debate Rages," *Chicago Tribune* (14 June 1987), Section 1, l).   A retired bank president, Stuart Dingle, entered Saint John's hospital in Detroit to clear the arteries of his heart. During the procedure his heart stopped; after being revived, his heart depended upon an external pacemaker to keep beating. Three cardiologists concurred that a pacemaker needed to be implanted in order for him to live, but the Medicare physician reviewer in this case denied all three recommendations.   The surgeon, Dr. Jacques Beaudoin, finally told the reviewer: "I'm sorry, I'll have to hang up. I've got to put this pacemaker in." Dingle, who had a long history of heart trouble, said of his case: "If they

had listened to Medicare, I'd probably have been dead." See: M. L. Millenson, "System Puts Doctors, Cost Cutters at Odds," *Chicago Tribune* (15 June 1987), Section 1, 1.

43. P. Lain-Entralgo, "What Does 'Good' Mean in Good Patient?" in *Changing Values in Medicine*, ed. Eric Cassell and Mark Siegler (Frederick, MD: University Publications of America, 1985), pp. 127ff.

44. Pellegrino and Thomasma, *For the Patient's Good*, last chapter.

45. Ibid., chapter 8.

46. Thomas Swick, "Experimental Cancer Clinic Grows and With It, Controversy" *American College of Physicians Observer* 7, no. 1 (January 1987), 1, 8-9.

47. Ibid.

48. Leonard Bailey, *et al.*, "Baboon-to-Human Cardiac Xenotransplantation in a Neonate," *Journal of the American Medical Association* 254, no. 23 (20 December 1985), 3321-3329.

49. "Chad Green," television transcript, "The Phil Donahue Show," November 16, 1979 (Cincinnati: Multimedia Productions, 1979).

50. *In re Bouvia*. Division 2, 2nd Civ. No. B 109134 (Super. Ct. No. C 583828) April 16, 1986, Court of Appeals of the State of California, Second Appellate, Division 2.

51. Joseph Fletcher, "Medical Resistance to the Right to Die."

52. Gene H. Stollerman, "Editorial: The Right to Serve and the Limits of Autonomy."

53. David C. Thomasma, "Editorial: Caveat Philosophus: Technology's Abuse-Potential in the Decision to Terminate Life."

54. It should be noted that we do not agree with this particular theory of organ retrieval. See Thomas O'Donnell, "Organ Transplantation," *Health Progress*; David C. Thomasma, "A Theological Perspective on Organ Transplantation," *Health Progress*, both forthcoming.

55. Loewy, *Ethical Dilemmas*, pp. 19-32.

56. David C. Thomasma, "Why Philosophers Should Offer Clinical Ethics Recommendations," *Proceedings of the National Meeting of the Society for Health and Human Values*, Toledo, OH, April 1987, forthcoming.

57. For example, the big bang theory has been worked out in quantum mechanical terms to such an extent that a debate was held in the spring of 1987 at the Fermi Lab outside Chicago on the possibility of God. Stephen Hawking was one of the participants. All were scientists. The reason for the debate stems from the fact that the universe behaved precisely in terms of the mathematical requirements of the laws of quantum mechanics at the critical point of 1/1 millionth of a second. Did the laws preexist the creation of the universe? Or were they inherent properties of matter itself originating with the big bang? Is an "Observer" or "Interpreter" necessary to the very behavior of this primitive matter?

58. H. Richard Niebuhr called these a "center of value." One would be conscientious towards such a center, or faithful to the set of values such a center represented. It can be argued, as Garrett does, that a religious view of life requires a radical relativizing of human life. See Paul Garrett, "The Center of Value in Medical Ethics: The Religious Context of the Practice of Medicine," paper read at the Annual National Convention of the American Academy of Religion, Chicago, IL, 9 December 1984.

59. David Barnard, "Meaning-Centered Medicine: Medical Ethics and the Study of Religion," Paper delivered at the Annual National Convention of the American Academy of Religion, Chicago, IL, 10 December 1984.

60. Ibid., p. 16.

61. Alan Donagan, A Theory of Morality (Chicago: University of Chicago Press, 1977), 61.

62. James Walter, "The Meaning and Validity of Quality of Life Judgments in Contemporary Roman Catholic Medical Ethics," Louvain Studies 13 (Fall 1988). Quote is from ms. p. 4.

63. J. M. Boyle, Jr., "Aquinas, Kant, and Donagan on Moral Principles," New Scholasticism 58 (Autumn 1984), p. 397.

64. John Ladd's interpretation of the context of personal relationships as inaugurating moral responsibilities is very close to our understanding of contexts as functioning moral rules. See his "Legalism and Medical Ethics," Journal of Medicine and Philosophy 4, no. 1 (March 1979), 70-80. Also interesting is the "prudential personalism" of Ashley and O'Rourke.

65. David C. Thomasma, Medical Ethics: A Case Studies Approach, Coursebook.

66. S. Bok, Lying: Moral Choice in Public and Private Life (New York: Random House, 1979).

67. Graber, Beasley, Eaddy, Ethical Analysis of Clinical Medicine, pp. 20-49.

APPENDIX A
Substantive Issues Discussed

CHAPTER

CHAPTER

CHAPTER

APPENDIX B
Strengths and Weaknesses of Models

STRENGTHS	WEAKNESSES

APPLICATION MODEL

▸ rigor, order ▸ acting on principle ▸ avoid relativism	▸ degenerates into legalism ▸ lacks sensitivity to context ▸ cannot weight fundamental moral principles ▸ ignores elements of context ▸ agreement on principles does not lead to agreement on conclusions

MEDIATION MODEL

▸ agreement in practice possible even when disagreeing in principle ▸ respects some relativity (cultural variations)	▸ muddle of induction and deduction ▸ no reconciliation of fundamental principles ▸ possible disputes about mediating principles ▸ Question: Does theory matter at all?

VALIDATION MODEL

▸ respect for descriptive data and disciplines ▸ respect for pluralism of principles ▸ broad appeal ▸ inductive checks ▸ action-orientation ▸ reconciling conflicting moral principles in a policy	▸ danger of naturalistic fallacy ▸ rule by experts

DETERMINATION MODEL

▸ clinically compatible ▸ respects contexts ▸ still a role for principles ▸ provides explicit means for prioritizing middle-level axioms, rules, and principles	▸ naturalistic fallacy ▸ loss of logical rigor ▸ danger of temporally or culturally determined or conditioned responses ▸ little respect for principles ▸ danger of reduction to what is currently in vogue in medicine (technology dependent)

STRENGTHS	WEAKNESSES

ORIGINATION MODEL

- ▶ respects diversity of values in medicine
- ▶ blend experience and precepts in the doctor-patient relation
- ▶ origins of axioms and principles from medical practice (avoidance of relativism)
- ▶ validation of goals of medicine as ethical
- ▶ "backdrop" as normative force (hidden assumptions)
- ▶ responsiveness to cultural change

- ▶ concrete can be too seductive - may sway reasonable policies or principles - poor link to theory
- ▶ can function as incorrect paradigm - naturalistic fallacy
- ▶ poor at dealing with community or preventive medicine
- ▶ contentlessness

VIRTUE MODEL

- ▶ compatible with codes of professional ethics
- ▶ death of human feelings, life, joys and tragedies
- ▶ discerning judgment and relativism

- ▶ cannot resolve moral disagreements (one's virtue is another's vice)
- ▶ requires independent principles or standards
- ▶ cannot be sole approach (not all problems are based on deficiencies of character)
- ▶ confuses moral character and professional traits

INDEX